Includes Four-Week Application Workbook

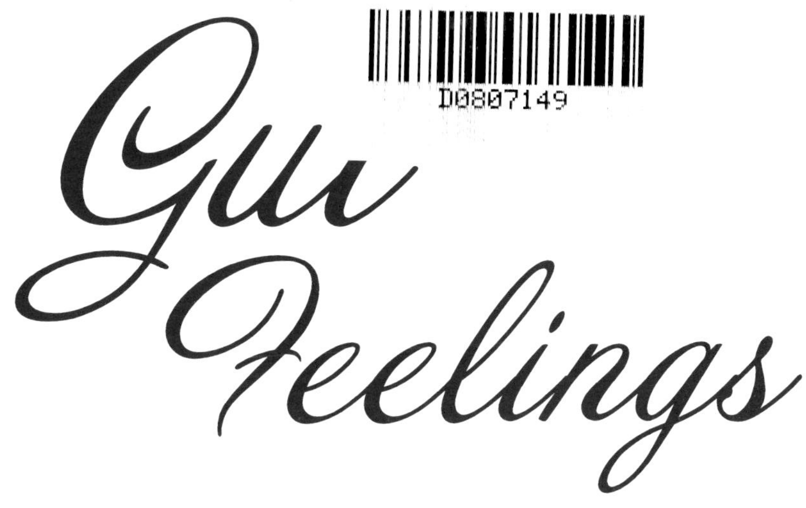

Unlocking Spiritual, Nutritional, & Intestinal Links to Anxiety, Depression, & Fatigue

Sharon R. Price, PhD., CN

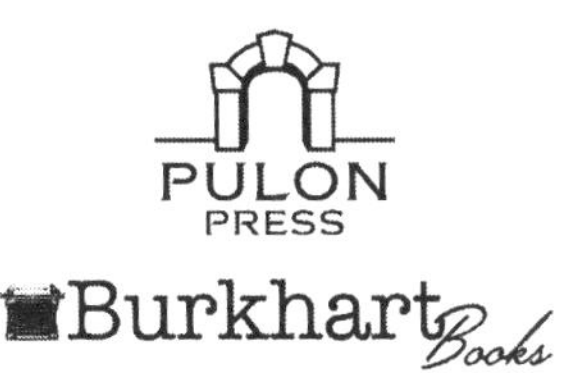

ISBN: 978-1-940359-43-4
Library of Congress Control Number: 2016958694

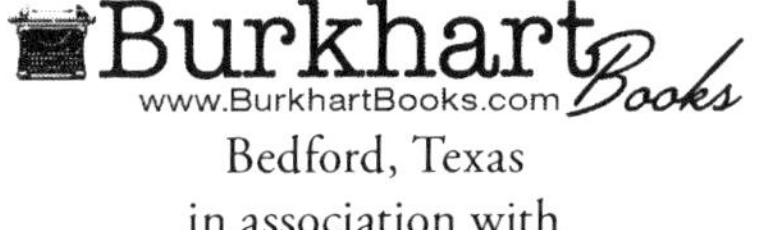

Bedford, Texas
in association with
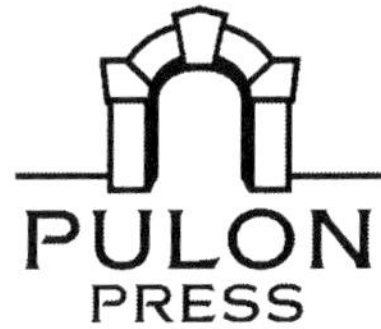

Dedication

To my precious granddaughters, Aubrey and Bailey—I never could've imagined the love and joy you bring to my life.

To their amazing daddy, my son, Justin. You are a rock to your family. As always, I pray that you witness Jesus name to millions.

To their remarkable mother and my daughter-in-law, Ryndi, who has diligently pursued and regained healing in her life. You are an inspiration.

And most of all, to God, my Creator and Father, in whom there is no variation or shifting shadow. You, O LORD, have shown me over the years that You are faithful and changeless. All the glory truly belongs to You.

Acknowledgments

I am eternally grateful to God who put me on a path of personal physical, emotional, and spiritual healing twenty-eight years ago, and then created the Ministry of Nutritional Direction to encourage others on a similar journey. All glory and honor belong to You.

I am grateful for my thousands of clients over the years who have placed their trust in me to help improve or regain their health. You have urged me on and challenged me to fit together the puzzle pieces of our amazing bodies.

I don't know how I would've been able to work through this book and bring it to a conclusion without all the encouragement and prayers from my family, my friends, and my clients. Without naming everyone, you know who you are.

I want to especially thank two treasured friends, Patty Balloun and Kara Diane Foster for reading my manuscript throughout the process and providing feedback. Also, I am grateful to my dear friend, Alexandra Christian, for taking time from her busy schedule to quickly edit my document. And all the others whose opinions helped to build this book.

DISCLAIMER: Information presented in this book and related workbook is intended only as a guide to those seeking a higher level of health. This information is not intended to diagnose, treat, heal, or cure. Words related to heal or healing are meant to be reflective of the body's innate divine-designed ability to heal. The author assumes no responsibility for any result of applying this information.

Contents

Part Five: The Role of Inflammation in Depression and Anxiety

Part Six: Restoring Mental and Emotional Health through the Gut Highway

Introduction

After writing my first book, Health and the Domino Effect in 2002, now out of print, I was excited about getting started on my next book. However, one day during my daily time with the Lord, I distinctly heard Him say to me, "Daughter, you don't know yet what I want you to write." Now, more than ten years later, the message that He wants me to send resonates in the pages of this book.

Over the last twenty plus years, I have had thousands of consultations with individuals, many whose chief and chronic complaints were depression, anxiety, and fatigue. Every single one of these clients also had some gastrointestinal distress. Around year five I discovered a pattern in most of these cases. These individuals became virtually symptom-free when they followed a strict protocol to return gut health to normal. Not only symptom-free but as the body was given the proper support to heal the underlying causes, these individuals were no longer burdened by issues of depression, anxiety, and fatigue, as long as they did not return to their original lifestyles.

While this may sound quite simple, to me it seemed profound, as though a dimmer switch in my brain had suddenly been turned to bright. I realized that I saw myself in these clients. Depression, exhaustion, and gastrointestinal issues worsened by life stressors were three of the main issues that got my attention and propelled me to seek help more than twenty-five years ago. You will find "My Own Journey," my brief personal testimony to the faithfulness of God, as the final chapter in this book.

As I began to interact with the local church women through speaking engagements, Bible studies, conferences, and women's groups, I also realized that anxiety, depression, and fatigue are very common in the church today, and at the very root of these symptoms are gastrointestinal tracts that are begging for help.

In addition to these physical and emotional issues, many of my clients, who also happened to be part of the local church body, were suffering from varying degrees of guilt, shame, rejection, pride, fear, bitterness, anger, and unforgiveness. Once again, I recognized myself in these precious clients. The research shows that twice as many women as men develop depression. These are very real issues for women who've had abortions, as well as men and women who have been victims of physical, emotional, sexual, or religious abuse. Many times these individuals are not even aware of the negative roots that create bondage in the believer. The bondage is spiritual, but in killing the joy of the soul, it will also affect the body mentally, emotionally, and physiologically. The physical and mental body cannot be well unless the spirit (soul) is free of these stifling bondages.

Those who are unaware of nutritional therapies and functional or forensic nutrition are helpless. I am called to take a stand for Jesus Christ, to break the strongholds of the enemy against those who are broken physically, emotionally, and spiritually. My goal in writing this book is that you will understand the intricate intertwining of physical, emotional, and spiritual health, and be blessed with peace and hope for your health just like my clients and I were.

Part One

Health the Way God Intended

Man and Machine

Before God called me to help others through nutritional therapies, I was in the corporate world and was identified as a "Filtration Product Sales Manager." My goals were, of course, based on how much product (hydraulic oil filters) I and my team of distributors sold. I became extremely knowledgeable about contamination from any source within a hydraulic system. I read and studied everything I could get my hands on and was amazed to learn that more than 90% of hydraulic equipment failures (pumps, motors, valves) result from "dirty" oil. In fact, we could predict just about when a failure would occur based on the cleanliness of the oil. I was excited! I felt like I had the 'secret' to saving companies hundreds of thousands and perhaps millions of dollars in hydraulic equipment repair costs, not to mention machine downtime.

I realized that if I could just educate the decision makers on the significance of clean oil, showing the research, I could convince them, or better yet, they could draw their own conclusions. These companies would then take a proactive, cause-effect analysis approach to machine maintenance and dramatically increase the health and life of their equipment. Some were convinced and immediately installed my brand of filters. Even after the initial expense of purchasing and installing these relatively high-priced oil filters, they realized thousands of dollars in savings. They reaped the rewards of identifying and fixing the cause of system failures. Others chose not to make changes and continued steeped in their costly ignorance.

Right about now you're probably thinking, "So, what does all this hydraulic stuff have to do with my health?" As I began to study nutrition, God gave me the amazing analogy of machine maintenance and its correlation to the 'maintenance' of our own bodies. A smooth and efficiently running body is directly related to the 'cleanliness' of our systems. An overburden of toxins will clog up the liver (the filter) and put a strain on all other organs and systems. Symptoms such as an increase in blood pressure, similar to the increase in machine hydraulic pressure; muscle and joint aches and pains like stressed and weakened hydraulic hoses from

Pain is a great motivator that the body uses to seek comfort or healing.

contamination, and intermittent headaches analogous to a sticking or leaking hydraulic valve, can all either be acted upon or ignored.

Unlike a hydraulic machine, God created your body in a miraculous way, which is to naturally seek healing. Pain is a great motivator that the body uses to seek comfort or healing. You can either do something about it or ignore it. The popular motivational speaker, Tony Robbins, once said, "Change happens when the pain of staying the same is greater than the pain of change." That phrase applies to simply repositioning your body after you sat on your legs too long. It also applies to a frightening cancer diagnosis after a routine colonoscopy. You either do something about it, or you ignore it.

Dr. Paul Brand, who died at age eighty-eight, was a medical doctor and a world-renowned hand surgeon and leprosy specialist. Dr. Brand worked with leprosy patients for almost twenty years in India, and co-wrote with Phillip Yancey the excellent book, In His Image. He wrote about leprosy patients whose skin had deteriorated from bacterial infection that destroyed their nerves. Their sense of touch was destroyed, and they feel no pain. Dr. Brand said, "A leprosy patient [has] lost this incessant hum of intercellular conversation." He says:

> "It would have been far easier and more pleasant for God simply to abolish pain rather than to share it. Pain exists not as a proof of God's lack of concern, but because it has a place in creation significant enough that it cannot be removed without great loss. I, of course, see the effects of that loss every day in my leprosy patients. For this reason, if I held in my hand the ability to eliminate human pain, I would not exercise the right. Pain's value is too great. Rather, I lend my energies to doing all I can to help when that pain turns into suffering."

We are so accustomed to and take for granted the God-designed phenomenon of pain that we rarely consider the body's amazing healing capability. For instance, when you cut your hand with a kitchen knife, enzymes and fibrin rush to the wound to coagulate the blood. Zinc, vitamin C, vitamin E, collagen, and other nutrients repair the skin so that no scar remains. Or, in the case of an epithelial tear in an artery, your body creates cholesterol to patch the tear.

Genesis, chapter 1, verse 27 states that "God created man in His own image, in the image of God He created him; male and female He created them." He is pure and perfect, and He created us in His image to be pure and perfect. However, as the first of God's human creation, Adam's sin of disobedience in the garden caused an imperfect nature in each one of us. But, because of God's incomparable grace and mercy we have the opportunity to conform once again to His image through His Son's shed blood on the cross. That is why Jesus came to earth. Oswald Chambers says in his time-honored devotional *My Utmost for His Highest*:

> "God nowhere holds a person responsible for having the heredity of sin [through Adam] and does not condemn anyone because of it. Condemnation comes when I realize that Jesus Christ came to deliver me from the heredity of sin, and yet I refuse to let Him do so."

Those who believe the following words spoken by Jesus in John 3:16 will have an eternally pure and perfect body.

> *For God so loved the world that He gave His only begotten Son, that whoever believes in Him shall not perish, but have eternal life.*

Your body must deal with variables on a constant basis to maintain homeostasis or balance—variables such as too little sleep, eating in excess, dehydration, negative emotions or attitudes, life stressors, environmental or chemical pollutants, and others. Once again, God designed the body to deal with these issues. The liver and kidneys were designed to convert and filter out environmental toxins and chemicals, including those caused by negative emotions. The adrenals were designed to protect and balance the body against stressors. And dehydration can signal the brain to "pass-out" the body to conserve energy until the trauma can be resolved.

But constantly burdening the body makes that adaptation more and more difficult. Have you ever heard anyone say or said yourself, "I haven't been sick a day in my life, and now suddenly I've been diagnosed with cancer"? Many 'suddenly' diagnosed illnesses are the result of what is called functional disease (also called sub-clinical)—a disease whose path has been littered with unhealthy choices and may not display obvious symptoms for perhaps many years. It's the one final unhealthy choice that broke the proverbial camel's back. Cancer and osteoporosis are two examples of diseases that have a functional or sub-clinical pattern.

Signals and Alarms

Think of homeostasis as a pendulum. If that pendulum swings within the parameters of centeredness, then your body will stay balanced and function properly within God's design for inherent healing. As the pendulum moves outside those parameters, it becomes compromised, unstable, and in need of attention. Depending on your genetic structure and biochemical make-up, your body will be forgiving of abuses for only a specified length of time.

Think back to when you first went off to college or got your first job or were on your own for the first time. Like me, you probably thought to yourself, "Yeah! Now I can do whatever I want, eat and drink when and whatever I please, sleep whenever I want, party all the time, and life will be good!" These are abuses that start the pendulum to swing outside of centeredness, and it continues that swing for months, maybe years. Through overuse, abuse, and excessive burden, your body depletes or damages its God-designed healing capabilities. Ignoring signals such as headaches, mood swings, brain fog, gas, bloating, reflux, constipation, or diarrhea, compromises your body's natural healing ability. If these signals are ignored, your body will sound alarms such as:

- Abdominal cramping requiring a visit to the emergency room
- Anxiety causing pain and heaviness in the chest
- Debilitating depression
- Overwhelming fatigue and exhaustion
- Body aches and pains

Listen to your body's many whispers and cries for help. These signals are the first warning signs of a body out of balance. First Peter 5:8 says, "Your adversary the devil prowls around like a roaring lion seeking someone to devour." Considering your state of health today, can you hear the enemy knocking on your door? The subtle signals mentioned above can easily be ignored. But signals allowed to escalate to the alarm phase will interfere not only with your ability to recognize the enemy but, also and more importantly, with your relationship with Jesus Christ. By the time your symptoms reach the alarm phase, the pendulum has become "stuck." Most individuals are forced to seek emergency treatment.

As you will read in the last chapter of this book, I became a believer in Jesus Christ about the same time I began to recognize that my physical and emotional health were spinning out of balance. I had ignored the subtle signals and was already in the alarm phase. During that period of my life, a sweet Christian lady named Karen who was my neighbor, taught me how important it is to recognize Satan's supernatural power and that of his minions. That knowledge gained from Karen

Listen to your body's many whispers and cries for help.

and through the Bible was a pivot point in my health journey. I learned to recognize the struggle for my body, mind, and soul and to find strength in knowing that greater is the Spirit of God Who is in me than the enemy who is in the world (1 John 4:4).

Satan doesn't always knock. He barges in uninvited, or we invite him in through open doors of unhealthy lifestyle choices, whether those choices are fast food, lack of exercise, addictions to alcohol, sugar, drugs (including prescription drug abuse), smoking, spiritual bondages, or an otherwise unbalanced life. And that is right where the enemy wants you!

A spiritual bondage or stronghold is a lie from the enemy that we have believed as truth either consciously or sub-consciously. It becomes a wall or a barrier preventing us from becoming all that God has created us to be. Such a stronghold might be shame and guilt heaped on by the enemy over the years. Other bondages might be unforgiveness, anger, or rejection—or lies that you're too fat, too skinny, too sick, not good enough, etc. The light of truth in the standard of God's word (the Bible) shines a light on these strongholds and exposes them for what they are—lies from the pit of hell, the home of the enemy of your soul. Do not allow him to keep that stronghold in your life. Recognize that God is greater and, if you are a believer, His Spirit resides in you, giving you the power to protect the miraculous healing power of your body.

Becoming familiar with your body is so important. You need not be an expert in anatomy or physiology to recognize the signs, signals, and symptoms that are your body's way of saying that all is not well. These signs and symptoms usually indicate functional illness and disease producing an imminent or developing failure of some physical or mental function. Every symptom is a God-given opportunity to find and fix what's wrong. Don't run from or ignore any of these afflictions, but instead, learn from them. Otherwise they become strongholds of the enemy.

Every symptom is a God-given opportunity to find and fix what's wrong.

Shelly Makes the Mind/Body Connection

Shelly (not her real name) says,

"You have been an enormous support physically and emotionally. There was a time that I thought all of my symptoms indicated a need for psychological help. To my relief, you have shown me that it was my body that was in need of rehabilitation. It was not my mind that I was losing, but my health. Thank you for listening to God's calling, thank you for going to all of those classes, thank you for sharing your knowledge with me."

Reversing Illness

To be discussed throughout this book, given the proper support, God created your body to heal itself. Your body strives for homeostasis, when all systems are working together properly. The sum total of a synergistically functioning body is more effective than each system working independently. However, your body systems do not work independently. Each requires input and feedback from the others, and no one body system is more important than another. Body systems and organs that become congested and toxic put stress and strain on other organs. Yet, as already stated, the human body is very resilient and adaptive. You might go years with improper nutrition and lifestyle before you start to notice the effects. Diseases associated with nutrition—and most diseases are—can take a long time to manifest. By the time disease sets in, the connection to nutrition and lifestyle is often confused and unclear.

I always told my clients that symptoms in the alarm phase are the last signs in the disease process. Just as importantly, even though symptoms are the first to abate, upon implementing nutritional therapies it does not mean that the root cause has been addressed. By the time symptoms have shown, diseases are deep into the cellular structure and take longer to heal than just eliminating symptoms.

Symptoms such as fatigue, depression, anxiety, headaches, obesity, chronic colds and flu, indigestion, yeast infections, inability to concentrate, asthma, allergies, bad breath, constipation, diarrhea, bloating, and gas all indicate imbalances that will lead to disease if not addressed properly. Almost all of these symptoms can be reversed without pharmacological intervention. I always tell my clients that because they have chosen to implement nutritional therapies, we won't know this side of heaven which diseases we prevented.

Diseases like cancer, diabetes, multiple sclerosis, fibromyalgia*, and other degenerative and autoimmune diseases have a pattern of progression that can be stopped and reversed by returning the body to a proper balance (remember how the pendulum swings) before the diagnosis is made.

**Fibromyalgia is not a diagnosis—more accurately, it is a name assigned to a collection of symptoms.*

Pharmaceutical Drugs

As in my case more than twenty-five years ago, the abdominal cramping and chronic yeast infections drove me to seek help the only places I knew, the emergency room and the physician's office. Physicians are taught to diagnose through testing, whether in-office palpation, presenting symptoms, or blood work. Once the diagnosis is made, they are also taught to prescribe pharmaceutical drugs to alleviate the symptoms. They might mention dietary intake or lifestyle. But, because nutrition has not been part of a traditional medical education, most physicians don't have the expertise to counsel in this area.

Eli Lilly, who founded Lilly Pharmaceutical, once said that a drug without toxic effects is no drug at all.

Using a prescription drug or over-the-counter Band-Aid approach to cover up a symptom is like killing the messenger for bringing the bad news. Treating the symptoms with drugs can suppress the body's natural response, inhibit healing, and drive the disease or illness deeper into the cellular structure of the body. An alternative is available for almost every prescription drug in existence. In very few cases, the pharmaceutical approach may be the best temporary solution, but in many others, pharmaceuticals may unnecessarily deposit toxins or interfere with the body's natural processes to treat symptoms that are easily alleviated with nutritional therapies. Eli Lilly, who founded Lilly Pharmaceutical, once said that a drug without toxic effects is no drug at all. Getting to the root cause is critically important, which in most cases is directly related to the health of the gastrointestinal tract.

You have a choice and responsibility in maintaining a most favorable state of health. You can choose to optimize your chances for better health by properly supporting the body's balance with whole, clean, fresh food, supplements, exercise, reducing stress, improving digestion and absorption, and reducing toxicity. These are some of the tools that will be discussed throughout this book to help you overcome and defeat anxiety, depression, and fatigue.

As the physical body heals, it remains critical to remember the spiritual implications of ill health, which will be discussed further. Bondages of all kinds were initiated in the Garden of Eden when Adam and Eve disobeyed God's command not to eat from the tree of the knowledge of good and evil. Disobedience enslaves; obedience brings freedom. For example, children who know the boundaries established by parents and other authority figures are more secure and happy, and consequently less fearful.

Part Two
Your Divine Chemistry Lab

Your Chemistry Lab

Let's delve a little deeper into understanding the body. Think of your body as a chemistry lab designed and created by a divine God. Every single thing you put into your body has a chemical effect whether you eat it, inhale it, think about it, or absorb it through the skin. Every one of your other senses, sight, hearing, smell, and touch, has an effect on your biochemistry, too. These biochemical reactions affect the body physically, emotionally, and mentally, potentially causing annoying symptoms that might include mood swings, anxiety, fatigue, hyperactivity, lack of focus, inability to concentrate, or cravings.

A September 2008 study in the *Journal of Experimental Medicine* revealed that the human gene remembers a sugar hit for two weeks. The study team also reported that a sugar hit causes cells to switch off God-designed genetic controls that protect the body against diabetes and heart disease. DNA makes up the intricate design of our physical bodies as well as our mental and emotional states. This excellent study focused on the genetic damage caused by high sugar intake.

An incredible amount of research has been done and is currently underway in the area of epigenetics. This term relates to any process in the body that alters a gene's expression without changing the underlying DNA sequence. Many diseases and conditions have already been linked to these epigenetic changes including some cancers, autism, heart disease, and obesity. Interestingly enough, research shows each of these factors affects, and is affected by, the gut microbiome (combined genetic material of microorganisms living in the human gut). Specific genes are responsible for protecting against these diseases; however, scientists have learned that foods can turn these genes on and off. In addition, prolonged poor eating habits could permanently alter your DNA.

Think of your body as a chemistry lab designed and created by a Divine God.

Substances other than foods can damage the DNA such as environmental pollutants,

When you feed your body, you are either building health or promoting disease.

additives, preservatives, colorings, chemical sweeteners, pesticides, mineral oil, plastics, pharmaceutical drugs, creams, lotions, potions, and "beauty" injections. Even negative thoughts and emotions can affect DNA. Scientists who study biomarkers for DNA damage have implicated diet and lifestyle, among others. It would make sense, then, that each generation could become sicker and sicker—in other words, infants born with an already high body burden of toxins.

When you feed your body, you are either building health or promoting disease. Long term poor food choices can usher in serious symptoms like panic attacks, suicidal thoughts, obsessive-compulsive behavior, social phobias, mental confusion, violence, and aggressiveness. The prevalence of many types of so-called degenerative mental or emotional diseases, including Alzheimer's and Parkinson's, is an expression of the cellular hunger present in various widespread states of malnutrition and toxicity.

A Gut Feeling

Gut is such an inconsequential word for such a critical part of all-encompassing good health. Scientifically, "gut" is the term for the alimentary canal (gastrointestinal tract) from the pyloric opening between the stomach and duodenum and the anus. But, for the purposes of this book, the gut will include the entire alimentary canal from the mouth to the anus. The entire gastrointestinal tract maintains a defensive posture in that it provides a barrier between itself and the internal environment of the rest of the body. It also provides surveillance through immune system tracking to determine the tolerance to all intestinal contents. As soon as it detects a substance as a foreign invader, the immune system (as an integral part of the gut) produces antibodies, which grab onto the invaders in an attempt to render them harmless.

Although the gastrointestinal tract is scientifically referred to include the stomach, small intestine, and large intestine, much-needed help comes from other organs and systems. Complete digestion and absorption are not possible without the help of the brain, liver, gallbladder, pancreas, spinal column, central nervous system, immune system, lymphatic system, and cardiovascular system. It is far more accurate to recognize that the entire body plays a part in digestion, absorption, and elimination.

Dysfunctions in the gut can be linked to virtually every disease including depression, anxiety, panic attacks, fatigue, chronic pain, and allergies, in addition to diseases that have an obvious relationship to the intestines such as diverticulitis, colitis, celiac, Crohn's, spastic colon, other irritable bowel diseases, and colorectal cancer.

These conditions are not only preventable, but in many cases can be reversed. I speak from personal experience because I was diagnosed with diverticulitis more than twenty-five years ago. I didn't eat salads because they made my gut hurt. But now a day without at least one salad or raw vegetable is very uncommon for me. By the grace and mercy of God, I have not suffered from any inflammatory bowel issues for more than twenty years. A scripture that I held onto during that time of intense healing was Genesis 41, verse 52, "God has made me fruitful in the land of my affliction." And surely, He has caused the healing and revelation to come to pass.

The Mouth, Sense of Taste, and Digestion

Most of us have heard the phrase, "you are what you eat." The more physiologically accurate phrase is, "you are what you eat, digest, absorb, and eliminate." Digestion begins in the mouth. Even as soon as you think about food or smell food, amylase and other enzymes in the mouth are being secreted as saliva increases.

"... you are what you eat, digest, absorb, and eliminate."

More than ten thousand taste buds reside on the tongue that signal the brain to process what and how you taste. Just as the senses in your fingers, the soles of your feet, and other parts of the body signal the brain to identify what you have touched, the tongue responds in a similar manner. Five types of receptors inhabit the tongue that sense all of the flavors that you taste. They are salt, sweet, bitter, sour, and umami. Umami is a taste receptor identified only recently and is best described as savory. Parmesan or other aged cheeses, MSG, and soy sauce, are detected by these taste receptors.

The Stomach

Food travels from the mouth through the esophagus to the stomach. The pH of the stomach should be approximately "1" on the pH scale, which is very acidic. A drop of stomach acid (hydrochloric acid or Hcl) can eat through the paint on your car. The interior of the stomach must be acidic to break down protein and carbohydrate, but also to have the ability to kill parasites or bacteria such as H. pylori, E. coli, salmonella and others common to our foodstuffs today.

The stomach itself is protected from its acidic terrain by a mucosal barrier. When this barrier becomes aggravated by a bacteria such as H. pylori, the acid can drill a hole through it forming an ulcer. This bacteria is becoming more and more prevalent today. The most common transfer route is through food and water infected with the bacteria. For example, restaurant food is easily contaminated when employees fail to wash their hands properly. Once ingested, this bacteria will form a self-protecting biofilm that makes it very difficult to eradicate. Biofilms are discussed more in the chapter on toxin sources.

Acid blockers are one of the most commonly used drugs in America, whether prescription or over-the-counter, for common symptoms such as heartburn and gastric-esophageal reflux disease (GERD). But, these are only symptoms of the deeper issues that need to be addressed in another way. There are rare cases when an individual produces too much stomach acid. But symptoms of what might be considered over-production are much the same as under-production.

If the stomach produces insufficient hydrochloric acid and lacks the enzyme and bile support from the liver, gallbladder, and pancreas to break down protein, carbohydrates, and fat, then the food contents will sit in the stomach longer than necessary and putrefy and ferment. This gaseous production will cause the valve from the stomach to the esophagus to open moving bile acids into the esophagus, causing GERD and heartburn. The valves of the entire intestinal tract will become unsynchronized which causes other problems like gas, belching, bloating, or cramping.

Proton pump inhibitors (PPI) and H2 blockers commonly prescribed for heartburn and GERD inhibit the absorption of Vitamin B12, which can cause pernicious anemia and also interfere with liver methylation. Methylation is one of the processes (pathways) in the liver that converts hormones and detoxifies the end-products of neurotransmitter metabolism, including dopamine, epinephrine, and histamine, and thereby is crucial in stabilizing mental and emotional issues. These are just a few examples of how drugs like Nexium, Tagamet, or Prilosec treat a symptom, and ignore the root cause, and actually promote disease and illness through nutrient deficiencies.

Proton pump inhibitors are also associated with dementia as noted in a study published in the August 2015 *European Archives of Psychiatry and Clinical Neuroscience*. "Patients receiving PPI medication had a significantly increased risk of any dementia." This should come as no surprise since all of the B-vitamins are critical to not only the methylation pathways but to the brain and central nervous system, as well.

What is Methylation?

In the summer of 1998, I read an extensive article in *Natural Medicine Journal* by Dr. Joseph Pizzorno and Dr. Michael Murray; both Bastyr University-trained naturopathic physicians, entitled "Detoxification: A Naturopathic Perspective." I was fascinated by their discussion of the enormous responsibility of the liver, including the methylation pathway, and began applying this information to help my clients reach a new level of health.

Methylation is one of many liver processes that detoxify, convert, and contribute to a wide range of critical body functions. Scientists consider methylation as a critical epigenetic process, interference with which leads to serious health implications, including mental and emotional dysfunction. At the same time, improving the function of this pathway can substantially improve overall health. Symptoms that this pathway may not be working might be irritability, mood swings, anxiety, fatigue, estrogen excess, or gallbladder issues. Other nutrients besides Vitamin B12 that are critical for this pathway to function properly, are methylated folic acid, vitamin B6, methionine, and choline, among others.

Methylation defects may contribute to major chronic conditions such as:

- Anxiety, depression, bipolar disorder, schizophrenia, and other mood and psychiatric disorders
- Fatigue
- Addictive behaviors
- Cardiovascular disease
- Cancer
- Diabetes
- Alzheimer's disease
- Seizures
- Autoimmune disorders
- Premature aging

- Infertility, miscarriage, and other pregnancy issues
- Autism and other neuro-spectrum disorders
- Lyme disease
- And many others

Problems with liver methylation can be identified through functional genetic testing. European health care has been performing these tests for many years and found that as many as 50% of Europeans have genetic defects (polymorphisms) in this function. Many people have a genetic SNP (single nucleotide polymorphism—a faulty gene from one or both parents) which interferes with proper methylation function.

The key function of the genes associated with the methylation pathway provides coding or information for the enzyme called MTHFR that converts folic acid to its active form, 5-methyltetrahydrofolate (5MTHF). If this critical enzyme is missing, proper metabolic conversion is impossible, causing or complicating the above chronic conditions.

Most of us think of complications affecting the brain when considering Alzheimer's disease. However, since depleted vitamin B12 prevents proper methylation in the liver pathway, it will also indirectly affect the brain with the potential for depression, fatigue, and anxiety. A by-product of the methylation cycle is an amino acid called homocysteine. If the presence of this chemical in the blood rises too high, it will affect long-term cognitive function. A study conducted in Baltimore of 1,140 individuals between the ages of fifty and seventy found that higher homocysteine levels were "associated with worse function across a broad range of cognitive domains." Oxford researchers found that test subjects who took vitamin B6, folic acid, and vitamin B12 not only reduced their homocysteine levels, but catapulted their cognitive test scores by up to 70%.

I recommend the following tests to determine how well a client's methylation pathway is working, because it is a risk factor for so many disease processes:

Homocysteine, serum. If elevated, it indicates risk for cardiovascular disease and stroke, as well as Parkinson's and other neurodegenerative diseases.

MMA (Methylmalonate), serum. Elevated level is an early indicator of vitamin B12 deficiency and risk for neurodegenerative diseases.

Vitamin B12, serum. Usually depleted with stomach problems. A level of 850-1200 pg/mL is optimal.

MCV (mean corpuscular volume) part of a CBC (complete blood count) can be a first indicator of folate or B12 deficiency.

MTHFR (methyltetrahydrofolate-reductase), cheek swab that identifies faulty gene for this enzyme which converts folic acid to the activated form, 5-MTHF.

COMT (catechol-o-methyl transferase) cheek swab which identifies faulty gene for this enzyme which is involved in neurotransmitter conversion.

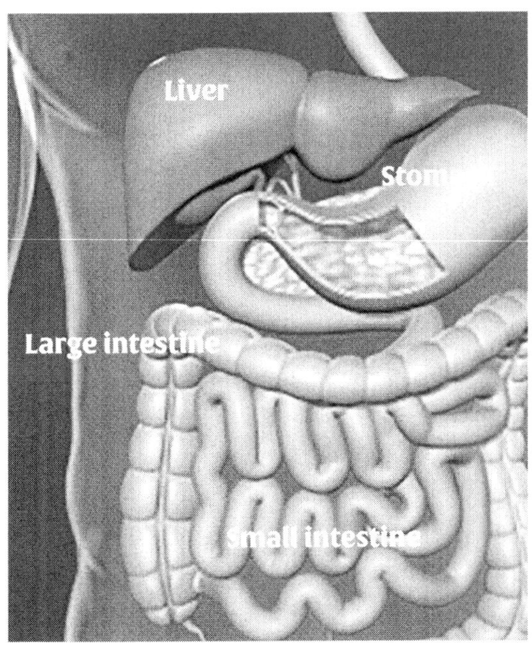

The Small Intestine

The small and large intestines comprise the largest terrain of the immune system. They are home to almost four pounds, or about one-hundred trillion and four-hundred different species of good and bad bacteria. Of the more common good bacteria, acidophilus strains reside in the small intestine and strains of bifidophilus bacteria reside in the large intestine. These bacteria must be balanced, are critical to the health of the gastrointestinal tract, and necessary to prevent almost every disease process. They synthesize vitamins, disable toxic materials, and are a key helper for the immune system. They also produce short chain fatty acids (SCFA's) from fiber that produce butyrate to protect intestinal permeability.

One of the main functions of these bacteria is to consume waste from the foods you eat. Think of one job of your intestines like your city sewer system. If you've ever taken a field trip to a raw sewage plant, you've seen the large tanks probably seventy-five feet in diameter and twenty feet deep. These tanks are filled with liquid (mostly water) into which sewage from our homes and businesses is pumped. The tanks are kept aerated and filled with bacteria, which consume the raw sewage to make it less toxic. Much the same thing happens in your intestinal tract. Balancing the bacteria that consume harmful materials is absolutely necessary for a fully functioning and healthy body. Research shows that disruption or depletion of these good bacteria contribute to dysbiosis (state of the GI tract that is a fertile ground for disease), and further interfere with delivery of information to the brain causing various mental health conditions such as anxiety, panic attacks, and depression.

Think of one job of your intestines like your city sewer system.

The small intestine is about twenty feet in length and about one inch in diameter. The pyloric sphincter valve from the terminal portion of the stomach opens up into the duodenum, the first part of the small intestine where most digestion occurs. Just as the stomach requires an acidic environment, the small intestine requires alkalinity for proper digestion and absorption. The brush-like border of the inner diameter of the small intestine called villi and microvilli are responsible for pulling the nutrients from the foods we eat. When these become damaged or destroyed through abuse, inflammation, or trauma malabsorption occurs which eventually leads to diagnoses such as Crohn's or celiac disease.

At the end of the small intestine, undigested or unabsorbed food enters the colon through the ileocecal valve. This valve is synchronized with the opening and closing of other valves throughout the GI tract, and like the other valves, this one can fail to function. Issues contributing to malfunction include the immune system response to food allergies, excess mucus, not enough water, and other inflammatory processes. This valve can temporarily be stuck either open or closed. If jammed in the open position, pathogenic bacteria from the large intestine travel backward into the small intestine, causing what is known as SIBO (small intestinal bacterial overgrowth). This disturbance creates inflammation causing anything from irritable bowel syndrome, bloating, and chronic abdominal pain to cystic fibrosis. The hydrogen and methane breath test is the only fully validated test for SIBO.

The Large Intestine

Many poor dietary choices, as well as stress, can cause the ileocecal valve to remain open, potentially causing SIBO, or get stuck closed causing constipation, bloating, or gas. The large intestine, also known as the bowel or colon, is the lower portion of the digestive tract and is about five feet long. A tubular shaped muscle, two and one-half inches in diameter, it can stretch enough to retain an extremely unhealthy twenty to twenty-five pounds of fecal matter. The healthy colon requires acidity for the final stages of nutrient absorption and to rid the body of undigested food and metabolic waste created by the liver and other body cells.

Material that was not digested in the small intestine is broken down by bacteria and may be absorbed. The healthy colon supports millions of various beneficial bacteria and other microscopic organisms. The principal bacteria in the colon, known as Bifidobacterium, synthesize vitamin K and produce some of the B vitamins. The transit time, or the time it takes between eating and eliminating the waste products from a food should take between eighteen and twenty-six hours. Less than twelve hours is too fast and not a long enough time period for proper absorption. More than twenty-six hours the waste begins to putrefy, ferment, and even cling to the intestinal wall. Imagine what would happen if you left your lunch on the sidewalk in Texas or Florida in 98.6-degree heat with 90 percent humidity for several days. The same result happens in your large intestine.

Damage and inflammation can occur throughout this entire length of the gastrointestinal, including destroying mucus where mucus should be or creating mucus where mucus should not be. Accumulated toxic waste, as well as bad bacteria, fungus, virus, and other pathogens, launch the process of functional disease causing signals or whispers for help such as constipation, diarrhea, gas, bloating, heartburn, GERD, and belching. If the process is ignored, then declining physical health is inevitable, including the soul sicknesses of anxiety, depression, and fatigue.

Part Three

What Causes a Toxic Body?

A Toxic Body

Have you ever moved after living in a home for many years? Junk gets stored in drawers, closets, garages, and places you forget about. What happens in the body over a period of years is very similar, especially when we ignore signals and alarms of malfunctioning. Harmful metabolites that aren't converted or removed from the body are stored in the joints, muscles, nerves, bones, etc.

Harmful metabolites that aren't converted or removed from the body get stored in the joints, muscles, nerves, bones, etc.

A toxic gastrointestinal tract is a favorable environment for parasites, fungus, yeast, bad bacteria, virus, and other organisms to build and prosper. As these organisms feast on the fermented and putrefied food end-products in the intestinal terrain, they create their own metabolic waste, which further burdens the body's detoxification processes.

Even if you ingest a good diet, you may still have more toxins than the body's systems can handle. We are exposed to foreign chemicals in our food, water, and air in the form of pesticides, antibiotics, herbicides, food coloring, additives, preservatives, hormones, nicotine, caffeine, and drugs. In addition, antibiotics, prescription and over-the-counter drugs place extra demands on the body, as well as contribute to an already toxic overload. Chemicals in the diet, as well as a poor diet, stress the liver, creating severe congestion, and compromise the body's main organ of detoxification. Further, a typical American diet does not contain sufficient nutrients to support the natural detoxification process.

Bowel Movements

Many people are not aware that less than one to three bowel movements a day is not normal. But the fact is, you should have at least one healthy bowel movement every day. Just as what goes up must come down, good digestion and absorption requires that what goes in must come out, less what is used for nutrition and energy. For the average American, the time for food to transit through the intestinal tract is an unhealthy ninety-six hours, as opposed to a healthful eighteen to twenty-six hours. The sluggish colon has an enormous capacity to collect waste. The collected waste, over time, rigidly attaches to the colon wall just like papier-mâché hardens, where it releases additional toxins and prevents proper nutrient absorption.

As waste putrefies in the GI tract instead of being properly digested, absorbed, or eliminated, the entire balance of the gut becomes displaced and confused. Poor diet, antibiotics, birth control pills, steroids, and a host of other physical and emotional stressors deplete the beneficial bacteria in the intestinal tract. These beneficial bacteria keep the harmful organisms in balance by taking up room, discouraging reproduction, eating some of the food supply, and otherwise fighting the harmful organisms. With inadequate beneficial bacteria, the harmful organisms are allowed to reproduce unchecked.

Other Body Burdens

Finally, detoxification cannot perform effectively when cholestasis, the liver's ability to clear stagnant bile through the ducts, is impaired. A healthy functioning liver and gallbladder are challenged by pregnancy, gallstones, alcohol abuse, anabolic steroids, and various chemicals or drugs, including birth control pills. One of the liver's key jobs, through its methylation pathway, is to convert and properly dismantle estrogen. Excess estrogen can cause cholestasis. In addition to estrogen, estrogen mimics, also called xenoestrogens, can be found in meats, dairy products, plastics, pollutants, pesticides, and body lotions and creams. These substances look like estrogen to the body, and the liver tries to process them as such, further burdening the detoxification process.

Lifestyle factors, such as not drinking enough purified water, can also stress the elimination process. Many years ago one of my mentors wisely said that the solution to pollution is dilution. Water is absolutely essential to all the body's functions. It makes up sixty to seventy percent of the body. Water is required to wash away metabolic waste, as well as to replace the loss of liquids that occurs every day. Stressors and a lack of exercise also affect the body's ability to detoxify. Exercise keeps the body parts and systems from getting sluggish. Stressors, on the other hand, have a way of tightening and impeding operation of the body's systems.

Exit Pathways

The elimination or exit pathways are key to carrying out the trash left over from every biochemical activity that takes place in the body. These exit pathways are the colon, kidneys, lymphatic system, respiratory system, and skin. Adequate nutrient precursors such as enzymes, amino acids, vitamins, and minerals are required to support this metabolic process.

The body's exit pathways can't perform effectively when more toxins must be eliminated than the nutrients and energy needed to perform detoxification and elimination. The nutrients may be missing from the diet, or they may not be absorbed properly. Toxic buildup can limit nutrient absorption, causing a vicious cycle to occur. For example, the body cannot detoxify heavy metals without the necessary vitamins, minerals, and amino acids. These toxic metals then take up residence in the tissues because they have no compulsion to leave. Excessive levels of lead, mercury, cadmium, aluminum, arsenic, and copper interfere with the normal functions of metabolic pathways and critical enzyme systems, further impairing the body's energy system.

Leaky-Gut Syndrome

Research overwhelmingly implicates "leaky-gut syndrome" and the resulting health issues of anxiety, depression, and fatigue. This particular aspect of gastrointestinal dysfunction refers to small and large intestine permeability or intestinal hyperpermeability. Complex protein structures called "tight junctions" are responsible for maintaining the seal of the entire intestinal tract. Fiber is a critical nutrient needed to make SCFA (short chain fatty acids) which in turn make butyrate to help seal these tight junctions.

In 2000, researchers at the University of Maryland, School of Medicine led by Alessio Fasano, found that these tight junctions loosen when a protein molecule called zonulin is activated by gliadin (a component of gluten in some grain products) or other food-derived triggers. The researchers further showed that increased zonulin creates inflammation and precedes the onset of autoimmune and other debilitating diseases, many of which include fatigue, anxiety, and depression.

This research concludes that autoimmune diseases start in the gut as the immune system creates antibodies directed against specific organs, causing tissue damage or loss of function. When these intestinal barriers are compromised, toxins and other microscopic substances like partially digested food particles, can penetrate the intestinal wall and leak into the bloodstream. These particles then circulate through the body and cause a number of symptoms, most notably food allergies and asthma. Moreover, gut permeability can cause the immune system itself to be confused and destroy the body's own cells, manifesting in any number of autoimmune diseases, such as rheumatoid arthritis, lupus, eczema, psoriasis, or Hashimoto's thyroiditis.

Complex protein structures called "tight junctions" are responsible for maintaining the seal of the entire intestinal tract.

Studies have also shown that intestinal permeability is responsible for chronic pediatric diseases, both mental and emotional. Foreign chemicals roaming through the body can alter RNA and DNA, the blueprint for cellular manufacturing. Alteration of these genetic structures can set the stage for cancer or other degenerative and autoimmune diseases, not to mention change to the genetic structure of future offspring. It certainly is no surprise, then, that disease states are becoming even more prevalent from generation to generation, disease states that struggle for diagnoses.

... disease states are becoming even more prevalent from generation to generation, disease states that struggle for diagnoses.

Various methods are available to determine if you are experiencing leaky gut. The easiest way is based on your symptoms. You likely have leaky gut if you suffer from fatigue, exhaustion, depression, or anxiety, coupled with any of the following:

- Chronic use of medications, aspirin, acetaminophen, NSAIDS, corticosteroids, or antibiotics
- Poor diet, including excessive alcohol
- Infections from parasites, virus, bacteria, or fungus
- Gut problems like GERD, IBS, IBD, gas, bloating, constipation, or diarrhea
- Food sensitivities, allergies, or asthma
- Chronic insomnia or sleeplessness
- Autoimmune diseases such as Hashimoto's thyroiditis, arthritis, etc.

Individuals affected by food sensitivities often find that leaky gut is to blame. Because of the onslaught of toxins that enter the bloodstream, the immune systems of people with intestinal hyperpermeability are on overdrive, mass-producing various antibodies. This, in turn, makes their bodies more susceptible to antigens in certain foods, especially gluten and dairy.

This list hardly excludes anyone, right? Take heart and continue reading; hope is straight ahead. Gut permeation can be healed, but it takes time, the right dietary intake, and the right cleansing and rebuilding programs. The right program varies for each person. No one program fits everyone. In January 2016, Owczarek, et al., concluded that, "It should also be remembered that there is no single common diet suitable for all IBD patients; each of them is unique and dietary recommendations must be individually developed for each patient, depending on the course of the disease, past surgical procedures, and type of pharmacotherapy."

While the body's organs and systems are always working to process toxins, the organs sometimes stop performing daily functions. Many symptoms of distress and disease can result from a buildup of toxins. Any quest for balanced physical and mental health can benefit enormously from extra support to these processes through diet, modified fasting, and other detoxification or cleansing methods which will be discussed in *Part Six, Restoring Mental and Emotional Health Through the Gut Highway.*

Sources of Toxic Burden

Generally speaking, a toxic body results from three basic causes: foreign pathogens, a body unprotected by balanced bacteria, and an inefficient detoxification system. This section will discuss the sources of those foreign pathogens, how they burden the body, how they contribute to anxiety, depression, and fatigue, and what you can do about them.

1. Antibiotics

Many medical doctors over-prescribe antibiotics. The treatment is quick, the pharmaceutical industry pushes it, insurance companies will pay for it, and many patients and parents request it. Antibiotics don't kill viruses, although many prescriptions are written for flu symptoms. In the past fifteen to twenty years, many new bacteria strains have become resistant to antibiotics.

Medical science and the pharmaceutical industry are scurrying to find a stronger antibiotic, one to which the general population is not resistant. Research is now showing that antibiotic resistance results from unhealthy biofilm complexes in our bodies made by these pathogenic invaders. These will be discussed in further detail later in this chapter.

Many children are born to mothers who are in the alarm phase of a functional disease or who are not able to breastfeed. Mothers' milk is very high in colostrum, a substance critical to stimulate an infant's immune system. Without this superior, God-designed defense, the prevalence of ear infections, ear tubes, pneumonia, colds, flu, pink eye, and other illnesses have become common.

Administering antibiotics year after year sets a child up and leaves the door wide open for a whole host of other illnesses, many of them serious. Antibiotics kill not only the bad bacteria but also the good, altering the balance of protective gut flora and immunity defense. The gut's immune system is disarmed, compromised, and incapable of defending the body against invasion.

Even adults give in to taking steroids orally or as an injection for pain and inflammation. In many cases, steroids are administered because antibiotics are not strong enough or they cause an allergic response. Steroids accomplish nothing more than temporarily alleviating inflammation and pain, putting the proverbial Band-Aid on the symptom, and pushing the symptom deeper into the body to surface later as a much worse condition. Some of the little-known side effects of routine steroid use are:

- Weight gain
- Serious fungal issues
- Stomach irritation or upset
- Glaucoma, cataracts

- Poor blood sugar regulation
- Thin skin and fragile bones
- Altered protein and carbohydrate metabolism
- Decreased absorption of calcium and phosphorous
- Fluid retention/edema
- Decreased resistance to infection

2. Fungal Overgrowth

A key result of antibiotic and steroid dosing is an overgrowth of yeast and fungus. Other causes of this pathogenic overgrowth are poor diet, including the consumption of dairy products and meat from cows and chickens injected with antibiotics. Birth control pills, immunosuppressant drugs, and too many stressors also contributor to fungal overgrowth. Fungus crowds out the beneficial bacteria in the intestines, which further drives the production of fungus. According to the Centers for Disease Control (CDC), over twenty species of candida yeasts can cause infection in humans, most notably candida albicans. This fungal species breaks down hyaluronic acid, which is a major building block of collagen and connective tissue. Research shows that candida is the most pathogenic fungus that threatens humans, causing a myriad of diseases and all manner of irritable bowel issues.

Neurotoxins

This neurotoxic genus of the fungi kingdom can grow anywhere in or on the body—lungs, fingernails, toenails, genitals of both women and men, oral cavity, and in the heart, causing mitral valve prolapse. As candida die off naturally or forcefully during a cleansing process, an endotoxin known as acetaldehyde is created. According to the International Agency for Research on Cancer of the World Health Organization (WHO), acetaldehyde is a highly toxic and mutagenic product that has been categorized as a Class I carcinogen for humans. The same toxic by-product is created when we drink alcohol in excess, resulting in a hangover.

As a result, you may experience brain fog or hangover symptoms as the breakdown of acetaldehyde occur and are carried out of the body. Acetaldehyde, a chemical breakdown byproduct of candida fungus, is toxic to the brain and central nervous system. It is no surprise, therefore, that this chemical is implicated in brain and central nervous system disorders such as anxiety, depression, and fatigue.

Acetaldehyde, a chemical breakdown byproduct of candida fungus, is toxic to the brain and central nervous system.

Acetaldehyde is also commonly used in manufacturing synthetic fragrances and a component of polluted air, tobacco smoke, and many foods. In addition to these toxic burdens, sugar feeds Candida and consequently causes sugar and carbohydrate cravings which will further exacerbate its growth and damaging side effects.

Some common symptoms or manifestations of candida and other fungal overgrowth are:

- Brain fog
- Sugar and carbohydrate cravings
- Fatigue, anxiety, and depression
- Vaginal yeast infection/jock itch
- Fingernail or toenail fungus
- Rashes, eczema, and other skin problems
- Chronic respiratory issues

During my physical and emotional trauma more than twenty-five years ago, the most overwhelming health issue that got my attention was chronic vaginal yeast infections. Of course, the physician gave me an anti-fungal prescription, Nizoral. I was unaware of the damaging side-effects that this drug could have on my liver but thankfully did not take it long. Neither was I informed of other options to deal with the root causes, such as dietary changes and natural remedies.

This and other chronic conditions propelled me on a path to discover the underlying causes. It proved to be a daunting task in those days before Google, *PubMed*, and all the other amazing internet options that are available today. Of course, considering the brain fog I had at that time, I would have been overwhelmed by all the information on the internet anyway. In those early days, I came across some poetry by Emily Dickinson, written in 1864, which came very close to describing how my brain felt:

I felt a cleaving in my mind
as if my brain had split.
I tried to match it seam by seam,
but could not make them fit.
The thought behind I strove to join
unto the thought before,
But sequence raveled out of sound
like balls upon a floor.

Pharmaceuticals such as Nystatin, Diflucan, and Nizoral are typical drugs used to kill fungus. Diflucan addresses yeast and fungus in the intestinal tract only, and Nystatin and Nizoral are prescribed for systemic fungus. They are all very difficult for the liver to process and liver function must be continually monitored with blood work. These drugs can also interfere with the liver's normal process of clearing and detoxification, and are useless to counteract the breakdown of chemical by-products of fungus like acetaldehyde, which can make one quite sick.

Much gentler yet effective natural remedies include caprylic acid, undecylenic acid, oregano oil, and grapefruit seed extract. An excellent probiotic with at least ten different strains of acidophilus and bifidus should also be added to repopulate the good bacteria, but should be taken at least four hours away from any pharmaceutical or natural antibacterials and antifungals. Supplements such as milk thistle and molybdenum will help the liver convert acetaldehyde into the less toxic acetic acid and remove it more efficiently. Xylitol is also very effective in inhibiting the enzyme that converts candida to acetaldehyde, especially in the oral cavity.

If you are experiencing brain fog, fatigue, or any mental issues like what I was experiencing, there is hope. Some health care professionals today believe that internal fungus is the root of all health problems, including cancer. While I respect and admire them tremendously, I am not focused on a singular cause of disease. I do believe that fungus and other pathogens need to be detoxed and expelled so the body can function again as God designed it.

3. Parasites

Parasites and fungus usually populate together and typically reside in the GI tract. But both can build a nest anywhere in the body. During my twenty plus years of counseling, I have seen clinical manifestations of how and where parasites exit the body. Parasites are very common in our civilized world and can come from food, water (drinking, swimming, and bathing), livestock, pets, walking barefoot, toilet seats, and travel to foreign countries. Symptoms of a parasitic infection may include:

- Rectal itching and pressure
- Diarrhea
- Mucus in stools and poorly formed stools
- Muscular wasting and weakness
- Chronic vague abdominal pain with constant belching
- Ravenous appetite
- Constant or frequent heartburn after eating

- Bloating after eating
- Digestive distress after eating fatty foods
- Unexplained weight loss or inability to gain weight
- Night sweats and insomnia
- Itchy skin, worse at night
- Chronic dark circles under the eyes
- Severe fatigue usually with a history of chronic anemia
- Unexplained nausea and vomiting
- Unexplained fever or chills

Many methods are available to eliminate parasites from the body. Metronidazole (Flagyl) is commonly prescribed by physicians to eradicate parasites and harmful bacteria. Herbs such as Artemisia absinthium (wormwood), garlic, clove bud essential oil, and black walnut hulls are very effective for eliminating parasites.

Biofilms

Candida and other fungi will never go away until parasites are expelled from the body. These parasitic and fungal pathogens, as well as virus and bacteria, are usually contained in a matrix known as biofilm. Biofilms research began in the late 1970s when Costerton and his colleagues began examining this gelatinous material. The Medical Dictionary defines biofilm as, "A thin layer of microorganisms adhering to the surface of a structure, which may be organic or inorganic, together with the polymers that they secrete." Another biologist describes biofilms as "... multicellular communities held together by a self-produced extracellular matrix." A good example of biofilm is dental plaque.

Candida and other fungi will never go away until parasites are expelled from the body.

The National Institutes of Health estimates that 60% of all human infections and 80% of infections unresponsive to medical treatment are attributable to biofilm colonies. In fact, these colonies can be a thousand times more resistant to antibiotics than bacteria that is not yet bound to a biofilm matrix.

Pathogens manufacture this jellylike material to ensure their survival, as well as to provide a hiding place for bacteria, virus, fungus, parasites, and even heavy metals. The tentacles of fungus, called hyphae, contribute to the biofilm matrix. They create another category of chronic infections that are extremely resistant to antibiotics. Biofilms gain momentum as the burden of pathogenic activity in the body increases. The biofilm creates, generates, and radiates inflammation. To release the burden on the body, biofilm must be shattered to destroy the pathogens contained in the slimy material. Further, unhealthy gut biofilm causes many different forms of GI distress and prevents the absorption of nutrients.

The biofilm is resistant to antibiotics. It is important to break open and destroy the biofilms. Natural herbal preparations that are most beneficial to destroy biofilms are a combination of enzymes called protease, cellulase, hemicellulose, and pectinase, any of which must be taken away from food. Ethylenediaminetetraacetic acid (EDTA) is also important to bind metals that contribute to the formation of biofilm. Biofilm busters should be used simultaneously with any of the previously mentioned antiparasitics, antifungals, and antibacterials.

Saccharomyces Boulardii has been shown to disrupt candida formation as well as biofilm formation. Curcumin has been researched and shown to be very effective in breaking up biofilms especially in relationship to fungus, virus, and bacteria. Although apple cider vinegar does not break up biofilm, it strips away minerals like calcium, magnesium, and iron, which contribute to their formation. Research shows xylitol, especially combined with ribose, is very effective to kill streptococcus bacteria and break up biofilms in the mouth.

Other effective agents in destroying unhealthy biofilms are:

- Propolis
- Cinnamon oil
- Quercetin
- Bismuth
- N-Acetyl-Cysteine
- Organic unrefined coconut oil
- Serrapeptase enzyme
- Reishi mushroom
- MCT (medium-chain triglyceride) oil

Although many forms of biofilms are unhealthy, they are not always a bad thing. Healthy biofilms are also formed by good bacteria. They create a thin mucus biofilm that is not inflammatory, but protective for the body. Good biofilms can exist throughout the entire body, including the mouth, esophagus, stomach, and intestines.

4. Virus and Bacteria

Virus and bad bacteria are other foreign invaders that compromise the terrain of the gut and the entire body. Already mentioned are helicobacter pylori, E.coli, salmonella, and streptococcus. According to the U.S. Department of Health and Human Services, bacteria that cause the most illness and hospitalization in the United States are salmonella, campylobacter, E. coli, listeria, and clostridium. Most of these bacteria are carried in food or water. Thousands upon thousands of other pathogenic and commensal bacteria can create imbalance, disease, and even death. The presence of bad bacteria is one of many reasons why the stomach must be acidic—to kill these bugs.

Virus and bacteria not only cause damage physically but mentally as well. Dr. Kazuhiro Kondo, of the Jikei University

School of Medicine in Japan, recently observed that the HHV-6 (human herpes virus) has been shown to cause mood disorders, most commonly major depression and bipolar disorder. This virus produces a rogue protein that increases calcium levels in brain tissues directly resulting in these psychological symptoms. This is just one example of a multitude of ways that virus and bacteria can cause damage, both physically and mentally.

Recent research into Alzheimer's disease has found that an amyloid plaque, a destructive biofilm in the brain, is a key reason for the disease. Research also found that the plaque formation in the brain is increased in the presence of latent herpes virus or other infections. The brain seems to be unusual in its relation to biofilms as it increases this biofilm (amyloid plaque) as a protective mechanism against harmful invaders. So, it's used as protection against virus, but at the same time increased biofilm plaque can cause Alzheimer's. Curcumin has been proven effective to destroy this plaque and further inhibit its formation.

Fungus, parasites, virus, bacteria, and their biofilms can also damage the gastrointestinal mucosal lining, another cause of intestinal hyperpermeability or leaky gut syndrome. As discussed previously, this can lead directly to food allergies, food sensitivities, or more serious diseases.

5. Heavy Metals, Phthalates, Parabens and Other Chemicals

Our world is bombarded with old and newly created harmful chemicals that surround us from the moment of conception. They're in our face cleansers, toothpaste, shower soap, shampoo, make-up, body lotions and potions, plastics, clothing, car materials, and furniture, not to mention the food we eat and the air we breathe. All of these chemicals interfere with our ability to keep our bodies healthy by burdening the immune system and upsetting the balance of detoxification. They also obstruct the body's divinely-orchestrated dance of hormones in the brain, organs and glands, and the central nervous system. Simply put, they burden the entire body.

The Environmental Working Group has developed a list of what they call the "Dirty Dozen Endocrine Disruptors." As you can see, the list includes three heavy metals.

- BPA
- Dioxin
- Atrazine
- Phthalates
- Perchlorate
- Fire retardants
- Lead
- Arsenic
- Mercury
- PFCs (perfluorinated chemicals)
- Organophosphate pesticides
- Glycol ethers

For the complete list with detailed information on why they are bad and how to avoid them, go to their website http://www.ewg.org/research/dirty-dozen-list-endocrine-disruptors.

6. Stressors

Stressors are also sources of toxins. It's not the stressor itself, but the thoughts we think about the stressor. The thoughts, whether negative or positive, about finances, jobs, time management, family or marriage, and social values all produce biochemical reactions that affect our health. Stressors are energy wasters and, as such, upset biochemical balance. Negative emotions relating to these stressors become part of the biochemical make-up of organs and systems.

Much research has been devoted to stress and its correlation to anxiety, depression, and gastrointestinal disorders—a definitive gut-brain connection—as well as gut-immune system interference. You will find more discussion on stress and its effect on the body in Part Four in the section on Adrenal Fatigue.

7. Poor Dietary Intake

Most people already know that dietary intake can be a huge source of toxic burden to the body. These toxic burdens include:

- Sugar
- Gluten
- Livestock treated with hormones and antibiotics
- Conventional milk and beef (with hormones and antibiotics)
- Chicken fed antibiotics
- Fish contaminated with mercury and other PCBs
- Farmed fish (common use of antibiotics and pesticides)
- Microwaved popcorn (bags are lined with harmful chemical)
- Rancid fats, vegetable oils, margarine aka plastic fat, fried foods
- Chemical sweeteners
- Genetically modified foods including soy, corn, and wheat
- Commercially grown foods (use of pesticides and low nutrient value)
- Additives, preservatives, and chemical colorings
- Sodas and diet sodas (chemical sweeteners, aluminum, and sugar)
- Peanuts, peanut butter, and corn containing aflatoxin (mold spores)
- High fructose corn syrup
- Agave syrup (processing creates high fructose levels)

The flavor and aroma of foods provide information to the body.

The flavor and aroma of foods provide information to the body. Many times, food characteristics provide protection to the body. For example, is the food rancid? But you cannot rely solely on flavor and aroma. Artificial sweeteners are chemicals added to food and drinks to mimic the taste of sugar, but with less food energy (calories). These are among the many fake foods that manufacturing companies' food scientists use to trick us into buying more and eating more. Most of the processed and packaged foods today are nutritionally void or at least nutritionally diluted. A key example of a fake food is a particular brand of dressings. I read that label ten times trying to determine how it could be manufactured as the label claims: "sugar-free, calorie-free, fat-free, carbohydrate-free, cholesterol-free, and gluten-free." How can their "Chocolate Syrup" not contain any calories, fat, carbohydrates, gluten or sugars of any kind? Chocolate/cocoa is naturally high in fat calories. In my opinion, these are bottles of water and chemicals, and I would suggest you run from them. These and other buzz words are marketing ploys to lull you into thinking you are doing a good thing for your health.

Part Four

Anxiety and Depression Are Not All in Your Head

Donuts and Road Rage: The Effect of Food on Mood

The American Automobile Association (AAAFoundation.org) says that most road rage occurs on sunny summer Fridays in moderately congested afternoon peak traffic. The time factor is very important here—at the end of a work day at the end of the week, when many people have fed themselves a nutrient depleted diet and experienced perhaps more than usual stress. A drop in blood sugar can be remedied not only by sugar, caffeine, and drugs but, unfortunately, also by aggressive and violent behaviors such as road rage, robbery, rape, or murder.

Let's take a look at what happens in your body's chemical laboratory when you eat. An entire cascade of biochemical reactions occurs. Valves open and close and practically every organ and system in the body becomes involved in breaking down food to create life-sustaining glucose for physical and mental energy. Glucose enters the bloodstream and, as blood sugar rises, the properly functioning pancreas releases insulin. Insulin, along with other enzymes and minerals from the stomach and liver, helps glucose exit the bloodstream and enter the cellular tissue. Some glucose is stored in the liver for later, on-demand access. Glucose is used as fuel for the body and the brain. When the glucose supply runs out, the God-designed body allows insulin levels to drop naturally.

If blood glucose gets too low, or the pancreas releases too much of the hormone insulin (hyperinsulinemia), hypoglycemia (low blood sugar) occurs. The body requires a very precise balance of glucose. Overindulgence in simple carbohydrates interferes with insulin and glucagon from the pancreas, eventually confusing the body's ability to receive and respond to the hormonal message, even if it was properly sent. Hormones are messages that require a recipient, or receptor site, to complete the cycle.

Hormones are messages that require a recipient, or receptor site, to complete the cycle.

Fasting blood sugar ranges are ideal between 60-90 mg/dl. When blood sugar drops below 50 mg/dl, hypoglycemia occurs resulting in a variety of strange symptoms that range from lethargy, irritability, and extreme weakness to anxiety and panic attacks. This is commonly observed in any office about three o'clock in the afternoon when half the office heads to the candy machine, the soda machine, or out for a smoke—anything to kick in the adrenals to release stored glucose from the liver to increase blood sugar levels

In a hypoglycemic state, the brain, or central processing unit, literally runs out of fuel. The body is in danger and can protect itself by becoming drowsy or sleepy. The adrenal hormones, adrenaline and cortisol—if functioning properly—kick in to convert stored glycogen in the liver to glucose. In the presence of adrenal fatigue or adrenal burnout, the adrenals are not able to respond properly. As a result, the body seeks quick remedies for sugar starvation by altering the brain.

Examples of quick, health-depleting remedies include donuts, candy bars, colas, coffee, cigarettes, cocaine, heroin, and other drugs. However, if these are unavailable, the body will do what's necessary to stimulate more glucose—hyperactivity, aggressiveness (as in road rage), or violence. Adrenaline itself, also known as epinephrine, can become an addictive substance. Ask any police officer, firefighter or first responder.

Neurotransmitters Role in Food and Mood

The human nervous system is made up of billions of neurons or nerve cells. Neurotransmitters, as part of the human nervous system, are the most rapid form of biochemical communication. Neurotransmitters are chemicals that communicate with each other and with other cells, like muscle cells, sending messages to various parts of the body. The primary neurotransmitters involved in all types of emotional issues are serotonin, dopamine, GABA, epinephrine, and norepinephrine. Secondary neurotransmitters that are affected by imbalances in the primary neurotransmitters, but just as important to emotional and mental issues are PEA (phenylethylamine), glutamate, and histamine.

Serotonin is found in small amounts in the brain. Recent research has shown that more than 90% of serotonin is produced in the gut to assist the enteric nervous system with digestion, making the health of the intestinal tract of crucial importance to re-balance all neurotransmitters. Serotonin is calming to the digestive tract, initiates peristalsis (contractions of the intestinal tract that move its contents forward) and secretory reflexes, and sends messages from the gut to the brain. Serotonin is also a mood stabilizer and regulates the sleep/wake cycle, appetite, and temperature.

Possible indicators of low serotonin:

- Anxiety or panic attacks
- Depression or bipolar disorder
- Poor digestion, including gas and bloating
- Carbohydrate and sugar cravings
- Headaches
- Insomnia
- Hot flashes

The endorphins known as dopamine, epinephrine, and norepinephrine are natural energizers. They are also involved in focus and concentration, motivation, anxiety, and sleep, as well as addictions and cravings.

Epinephrine is also known as adrenaline and will result in increased heart rate during the "fight or flight" adrenal response. It is also used medicinally as a stimulator after cardiac arrest or anaphylaxis (allergy reaction). Elevated norepinephrine and epinephrine levels will interfere with sleep and contribute to anxiety. Both of these neurotransmitters are also important for focus and concentration, energy and motivation, and to burn fat.

Dopamine is the upstream (precursor) neurotransmitter to norepinephrine and epinephrine. In other words, dopamine makes norepinephrine and epinephrine. Low levels of dopamine are responsible for addictions and cravings of all kinds, and high levels can be implicated in gastrointestinal issues. Dopamine is synthesized in the body mainly by nervous tissue and the medulla of the adrenal glands. Dopamine helps to regulate motor activity, motivation, attention, learning, and sleep.

Possible indicators of low dopamine:

- Addictions and cravings
- Lethargy or fatigue
- Sleeping too much
- Feelings of immobility
- Lack of motivation
- Procrastination

GABA is a natural sedative. Imbalances (either too high or too low) of this calming neurotransmitter will result in varying degrees of hyperactivity, anxiety, and sleep difficulties. GABA's primary function is to diminish the effects of excessive excitatory endorphins—dopamine, norepinephrine, and epinephrine.

Proper nutrition including vitamins, minerals, probiotics, and especially the building block amino acids from protein in the diet are instrumental in helping to restore neurotransmitter function. When minerals become depleted over long periods of time, neurotransmitters become unbalanced. In addition to proper diet, unbalanced neurotransmitters require targeted amino acid therapy guided by a qualified health care practitioner. Each neurotransmitter requires different combinations of these nutrients to rebalance the body's chemistry. Especially implicated in low levels of serotonin and dopamine production are stress (elevated cortisol levels), magnesium, zinc, and vitamin B6 deficiency, caffeine, sugar, and poor gut health.

Neurotransmitters help us to stay calm, happy, energized, focused, alert, and well rested. In other words, they support the body's subsequent adaptive responses. Ways to support this adaptive response will be discussed further in Part Six, Rebuilding with Micro-Nutrient Supplementation in the segment on Amino Acids.

From Miserable to Richly Blessed

Twenty-two-year-old Susanna (not her real name) says:

"I used to be a miserable product of my past. I had four different physical ailments that tormented me—depression, anxiety, lack of energy, and IBS ailments. I had an overwhelming slew of emotions that dragged me down to such a level that it was hard for me to get up to do anything at all. I had no idea that nutrition had anything to do with it. Furthermore, I thought that I was eating healthy.

"Then my mom helped me find Dr. Price who told me that depression and anxiety were common links to IBS. No one had told me that before. In fact, up until that point, I thought that IBS was a disease I was diagnosed with and that it would never go away. The medications alone were not healing me—I was still emotionally sick and physically undernourished. Now, with eating the right kinds of healthy food for my body, I have found a relief that even a year ago I did not know was possible. What's more is that through my gut being healed, the depression has also completely lifted. I realize that God has made our bodies in such a way that they mend themselves given the adequate support. Even sugar cravings had made me feel like a mere slave to my body—now I feel like I am its master, and rightly so! I am truly and richly blessed."

Sharon R. Price, PhD., CN

The Role of Adrenal Fatigue in Anxiety and Depression

When I began my nutritional practice in the 1990s, I continued to work on my Doctorate in Nutrition and Natural Health Science. I became fascinated with the adrenal glands partly because I was astounded at how my own health improved when I focused on adrenal recovery. The adrenals became the focus of my dissertation, "The Pathophysiology of Stress, Adrenal Activity, and the Causal Chain of Body Weight Dysfunction in Women." Even though my dissertation focused on weight in women and adrenal health, it continues to be an important part of the whole puzzle in helping individuals regain their health from fatigue, anxiety, and depression.

The natural hormones insulin (produced by the pancreas) and cortisol (produced by the adrenals) are the two most aging biochemicals in the body when continuously produced in excess. Cortisol is a secondary adrenal hormonal response, after adrenaline (epinephrine), when faced with chronic, unmanaged stressors. Overproduction of cortisol affects the ability of the pancreas to regulate blood sugar and results in unstable insulin levels, which lead to weight gain, especially around the mid-section.

Overproduction of these same hormones prevents the body from mounting a proper anti-inflammatory response and interferes with the capacity of the immune system to respond properly. By creating inflammation, these imbalanced hormones affect the integrity of the gastrointestinal tract by breaking down its protective mucosal barrier allowing toxins to circulate throughout the body. So many symptoms of ill health can be traced directly to adrenal function.

So many symptoms of ill health can be directly traced back to adrenal function.

The most common health complaints addressed in doctors' offices today include digestive problems, fatigue, depression, anxiety, and respiratory conditions. Often, the only remedies offered by the physician for these symptoms are pharmaceutical drugs such as Prozac, Xanax, Prevacid, inhalers, nebulizers, and bronchodilators. These drugs will never cure the underlying problem which, in many cases, is related to the adrenal glands. Moreover, they will interfere with the body's valiant attempt to heal itself.

What Are Adrenal Glands and What Do They Do?

Two adrenal glands each about the size of a walnut curve over the top of each kidney. Ad means "on top of" and renal refers to "kidney." The adrenals are an extremely important part of the entire hormonal system. The inner and outer layers of these glands produce hormones that help to maintain homeostasis. The glands are very small, but they carry out an enormous responsibility.

- The inner layer—the adrenal medulla—produces the hormones (also called by three other names—endorphins, catecholamines, or neurotransmitters) norepinephrine, epinephrine, and small amounts of dopamine. They are part of the sympathetic nervous system and responsible for the fight-or-flight response.

- The outer layer—the adrenal cortex—produces the sex hormones DHEA, pregnenolone, progesterone, estrogen, and testosterone and are involved in tissue repair, body rebuilding, and anti-aging. They are a backup system for the ovaries and testes.

- The outer layer also produces cortisol and glucocorticoids, which contribute significantly to blood sugar regulation, immune response, and anti-inflammatory actions.

- Other hormones produced by the outer layer include aldosterone and mineralocorticoids which regulate sodium, potassium, and fluid volume, as well as inflammation.

In recent years cortisol, a primary hormone produced by the adrenals, has been disparaged as a "bad" hormone. Nothing could be farther from the truth. Cortisol is critical to life, playing the starring role in the body's stress response. Cortisol does become an issue, however, when it is forced to work overtime and results in imbalanced health.

Potential sources of stress that increase an unhealthy demand for cortisol:

- Inability to properly digest and absorb foods
- Whiplash and other head trauma
- Inflammation and pain
- Prolonged temperature extremes
- Toxic exposures
- Infections
- Chemicals and radiation
- Negative emotions like anger, guilt, shame, worry, or fear
- Anxiety and depression
- Workaholism
- Sleep deprivation

The Adrenals Communicate with the Brain

God did not design your body to deal with constant stress. As with all hormones in the body, there is a rhythmic, divinely-designed ebb and flow that helps to maintain health. Dr. Hans Selye was an early pioneer in stress research. He discovered a relationship between stress and how the body responds. The hypothalamus gland in the skull stimulates the pituitary gland (also in the skull) to secrete hormones that synchronize the endocrine system. The adrenal glands are integral to this hypothalamus-pituitary-adrenal axis and release hormones called corticosteroids. Cortisol is one of these corticosteroids.

This circadian rhythm is maintained by the hypothalamic-pituitary-adrenal axis. The HPA axis is a beautiful example of the interweaving of two systems of the body, in this case, the central nervous system and the hormonal system—also called the neuroendocrine system. As resilient as the HPA axis might be, stressful or threatening situations throughout the day cause cortisol to surge and override it.

Over time, this phase of chronically elevated cortisol will manifest symptoms such as anxiety, panic attacks, fatigue, and depression, especially in the presence of digestive issues and neurotransmitter imbalance. If this phase of poor health is ignored, your body will remain in the exhaustion phase of adrenal stress response. Dr. Selye found that elevated levels of cortisol suppress the immune system by inhibiting beneficial pathogen-fighting T-cells and reducing the effectiveness of interferon, which kills viral invaders. Blood sugar balance, intestinal mucosal integrity, and emotional and mental function are also affected.

In a healthy person, cortisol should be at its lowest level around 9 PM. During sleep, cortisol production begins to climb again to its highest level around 6 AM. During the healthy cycles of light sleep, deeper slow-wave sleep, and REM sleep, your body regenerates and maintains cell repair and restores immune system function, among other maintenance activities. The chronically stressed person cannot adequately accomplish these maintenance and repair functions.

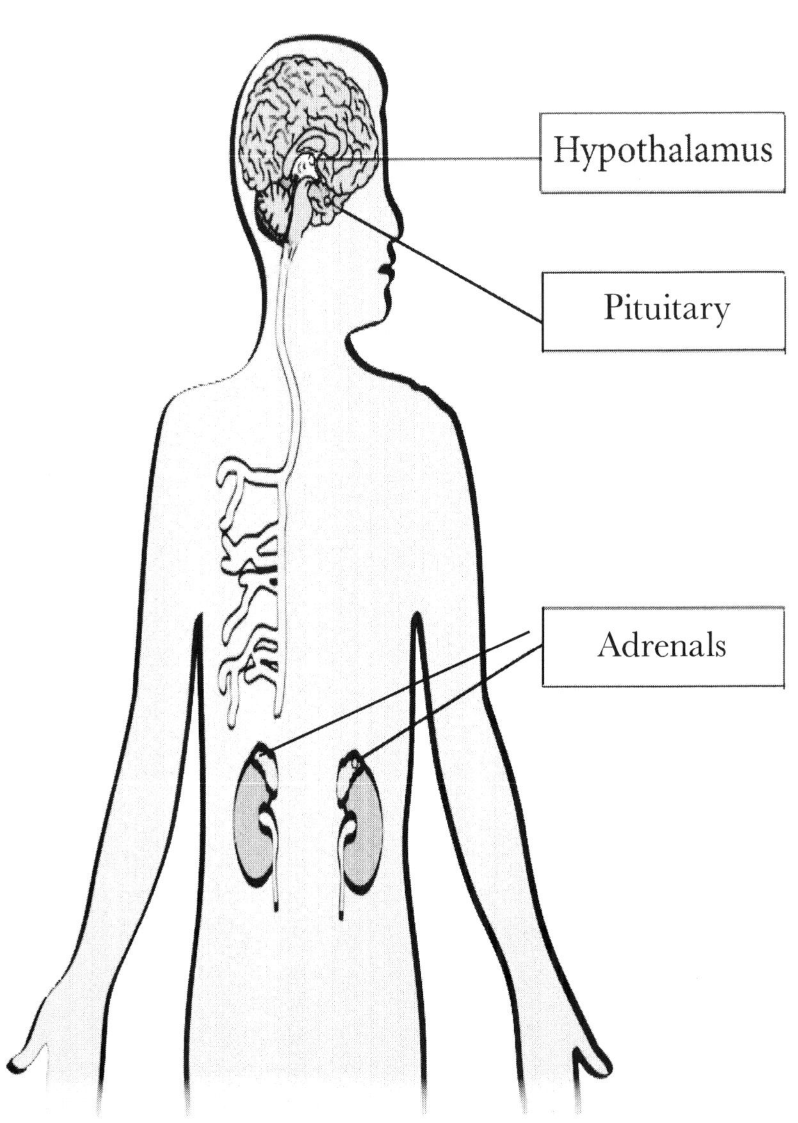
Hypothalamus
Pituitary
Adrenals

Your Body's Cascade Response to Stress

Dr. Selye discovered during his research that, regardless of the stressor, the body reacts with what he called a general adaptation syndrome. This syndrome manifests in three phases: the alarm reaction, the resistance stage, and the exhaustion stage.

The ***alarm reaction*** is synonymous with fight or flight—the body prepares itself to take action. The brain and pituitary gland respond by releasing adrenocorticotropic hormone (ACTH). This stimulates the adrenal glands to increase production of catecholamines epinephrine, norepinephrine, and cortisol. These, in turn, stimulate the heart to increase blood pressure and heart rate, while simultaneously constricting certain blood vessels to increase blood flow to the muscles and brain and decreasing it to the digestive tract and internal organs. This is why eating while in a stressful situation doesn't make good sense.

During the ***resistance stage,*** the body attempts to adapt to the stress. For example, the body begins to crave very high fat and simple carbohydrate foods to balance out anti-stress chemicals. Another biochemical response is increased glucose production which stimulates the fat enzyme, lipoprotein lipase, and causes excess stored body fat. To compound the problem, the excessive release of cortisol also impairs the body's ability to burn fat by disengaging a natural fat-burning enzyme called delta-6-denaturase. A shortage of this enzyme makes losing weight much more difficult therefore is associated with obesity.

At the same time, this rush of cortisol stimulates the liver to produce and release more glucose and cholesterol into the blood for energy. This stage of resistance can continue for a long time. Extended periods of stress during this stage can increase cholesterol levels, create a perfect environment for diabetes, and compromise immune function.

Finally, the body enters the ***exhaustion stage*** and begins to break down or metabolize stress hormones. Eventually, the body

Chronically high cortisol output by the adrenals will eventually result in adrenal burnout with symptoms including exhaustion, cognitive dysfunction, anxiety, and depression.

returns to normal, and a calming effect is experienced. According to Selye, these three stages can occur within seconds or take days, weeks, or even months, depending on the number and duration of stressors. Chronically high cortisol output will eventually result in adrenal burnout with symptoms including exhaustion, cognitive dysfunction, anxiety, and depression.

Dr. Archibald Hart, a clinical psychologist, made the best analogy I have heard for how stress can damage the body:

> "The clearest way I can illustrate this is to ask you to imagine an elastic band. If it is stretched between your thumbs and then quickly released, it easily returns to its normal, relaxed position. The body's stress response is also "stretched" whenever it is subjected to an emergency or demand. It ought to return to a normal, relaxed state when the emergency is over. But if the elastic band is stretched and then held in an extended position for a long period of time, it begins to lose its elastic properties and does not return to its former relaxed state. It develops hairline cracks and will eventually snap."

Even the slightest strain on the body through mental and physical stressors cause it to consume vitamins and minerals in excess of its normal needs. A sudden scare, an argument, or a slight cut or bruise all call on the body's special reserves. Dr. Selye found in his research on stress that if you inflict the same stressor on two different people, one malnourished and the other well-fed, the well-fed person adapts to the stress much better than the other.

Studies of the brain have shown that repetitive stressors and consequential increased cortisol levels cause inflammation in the hippocampal region of the brain and even damage or kill related cellular tissue. The hippocampus is essential for memory and learning and is dense with cortisol receptors. It is important to note that the hormone messaging cycle is only successful if the hormone being sent is properly received. If these receptor sites become damaged and, therefore, unable to receive the message, the cycle has been disrupted. It's like someone frantically calling to tell you that your house is burning down but you can't hear because you're sleeping, your music is too loud, or you've already passed out from the smoke. Receiving the message is critical. The ability of the hippocampus receptors to receive hormonal messages has been implicated in short-term memory recall, as well as changes in mood and behavior.

When burnout is critical the energy-producing systems of the body, primarily the adrenal glands and the thyroid, are severely compromised.

What is Adrenal Burn-Out?

Adrenal burnout is always preceded by chronic and ongoing adrenal fatigue. The fatigue derives from internal or external stressors triggering chronically elevated cortisol levels. The adrenals are functioning as God designed them, but become overworked and are unable to continue producing sufficient cortisol when needed, resulting in burnout. Inadequate adrenal function was first described in the literature over one-hundred years ago, calling it "hypoadrenia" (low adrenal). Dr. James L. Wilson renamed the syndrome Adrenal Fatigue in 1998 in his book *Adrenal Fatigue, The 21st Century Stress Syndrome.*

Burnout from adrenal fatigue can occur in varying degrees of severity. When burnout is critical, the body's energy-producing systems, primarily the adrenal glands and thyroid, are severely compromised. It might even be called a crash and burn syndrome, and it has far-reaching effects on the entire body. The body is unable to function normally to maintain balance. Distressing symptoms begin to appear, or present symptoms are magnified. Adrenal burnout differs from adrenal fatigue because getting more sleep will not cure it.

Common symptoms of adrenal burnout include brain fog, sleepiness, lethargy, shakiness, extreme weakness, anger, and irritability. These symptoms are identical to the symptoms of hypoglycemia (low blood sugar) or hyperinsulinemia (the pancreas secretes too much insulin). Therefore, restoring adrenal function is necessary to properly regulate blood sugar.

The effects of adrenal burnout are devastating for the individual and often for family and friends. The principal physical symptom that initially identifies burnout is overwhelming fatigue upon awakening in the morning or after a brief nap. The individual still feels exhausted. As one who suffered both forms, I would like to create a distinction between adrenal fatigue and adrenal burnout.

Biochemical changes that take place during ***adrenal fatigue***:

- Increased adrenaline
- Increased cortisol
- Loss of key minerals like magnesium, calcium, and potassium
- Carbohydrate/sugar malabsorption
- Thyroid suppression
- Increased blood sugar
- Bone loss
- Inability to break down protein

Symptoms of ***adrenal fatigue***:

- Increased allergies
- Bone pain
- Loss of lean muscle mass

- Recurring infections
- Sugar/carbohydrate cravings
- Obesity
- Irritability or moodiness
- Fluid retention
- Weight and fat gain around middle
- Impaired immune function

Biochemical changes during ***adrenal burnout***:

- Adrenaline depletion
- Insufficient cortisol response
- Depletion of progesterone, testosterone, and other hormones
- Decreased cellular energy
- Protein and fat malabsorption
- Decreased lean muscle mass
- HPA axis interference
- Depleted immune system
- Insulin resistance
- Inability to overcome inflammation
- Loss/damage of hippocampus receptors

Symptoms of ***adrenal burnout***:

- Poor memory or concentration
- Foggy thoughts
- Depression
- Anxiety and worry
- Feelings of guilt or shame
- Exhaustion
- Sense of being overwhelmed
- Insomnia or poor sleep
- Headaches

- Heart palpitation
- Low libido
- Cold hands and feet
- Chronic low blood pressure
- Back pain or tight neck and shoulders
- Muscle twitching
- Digestive/bowel issues
- Chronic infections, including skin rashes

How Adrenal Burnout Causes Depression & Anxiety

Toddlers and children suffer burnout as well. Heavy metals, food chemicals and additives, and other environmental pollutants all contribute to burnout at any age. These substances travel from the mother to the fetus through the placenta creating a perfect environment for adrenal burnout in the child.

Sadly, four out of five children and teenagers that I have counseled suffer from exhaustion and adrenal burnout. Burnout not only affects the physical body, but it also affects the individual mentally, emotionally, and spiritually. Teenage suicide rate has reached an alarming level—depression being a primary motivator. If the body is not functioning properly physically with support from the adrenals and thyroid energy-producing glands, it will naturally begin to shut itself down mentally to compensate and preserve itself. Suicide is the second leading cause of death for children and youth ages ten to twenty-four. More teenagers and young adults die from suicide than from cancer, heart disease, AIDS, birth defects, stroke, pneumonia, influenza, and chronic lung disease, combined.

Many children and teenagers are prescribed anti-anxiety medications as well as antidepressants. In addition to attending school, many teenagers work part time, play sports, and participate in extracurricular activities. Peer pressure and bullying hit harder with each generation. Children become anxious and wake up with stomach aches for fear of returning to school. And with parents being too busy to cook healthy meals, these teenagers become star performers in a nation of fast-food junkies. Depletion of critical nutrients interferes with cellular energy and neurotransmitter firing. If the child or young adult experiences difficult circumstances with the mindset of hopelessness and powerlessness, their spirit spirals down and sees the only way out as ending his life.

Burnout victims are usually hard driving, busy workaholics who refuse to stop for fear they will not be able to get up again.

A full 40-50% of my adult clients are in adrenal burnout as confirmed through hair analysis or saliva cortisol testing. These people do not lie around all day, even though they are exhausted. Their subconscious motto is "no guts, no glory." Many of them are exercising vigorously five or six times a week, hoping to get past the wall to increased energy levels. Long and difficult workouts are not good and will not only delay recovery from burnout but can make it worse. Burnout victims are usually hard driving, busy workaholics who refuse to stop for fear they will not be able to get up again.

Women, as caretakers and nurturers, often feel pressure or the need to say yes. They volunteer at school, at church, and in the community. They feel guilty if they don't exercise or work out at the gym. And they feel guilty when no energy is left at the end of the day for private time or lovemaking with their husband or spending time with friends.

Burnout does not occur overnight. It occurs gradually, over a period of time, relative to the individual's biochemical makeup and genetic structure. Some develop it quickly, others may never develop it, depending on what action is taken to prevent it. A combination of stressors over an individual's lifespan, exacerbated by an inadequate diet are the most direct causes.

This information may be depressing, but the purpose of this book is intended to bring hope and to discover the way out of adrenal fatigue/burnout, anxiety, and depression. God showed me the way out over twenty-five years ago. But, the enemy hasn't forgotten about my weaknesses and still tries to discourage me in that area. I know which food triggers depression for me, and I know what thoughts cause me to spiral down. I know what to do to keep my adrenals strong—if I'm paying attention.

Nutrient Depletion

Someone recently showed me that 'desserts' spelled backward is 'stressed.' I laughed because as a nutritionist I know that stress can cause cravings for sugar. The reverse is also true—too much sugar creates stressful deficiencies and imbalances in the body. Chocolate becomes the perfect food for someone in adrenal burnout because it contains many necessary nutrients which are lost during burnout. Chocolate contains theobromine and sugar, both stimulants, which are a welcome relief for someone who is exhausted or depressed.

As a consequence of adrenal burnout, the body must contend with thousands and thousands of different natural physiological and biological chemicals and hormones during these stressful episodes. During stressful times, the body has a high demand for magnesium, vitamin C, all the B vitamins, zinc, chromium, sodium, and potassium. These are always the first to be depleted, and in what order depends on the biochemical make-up of the individual. The body depletes essential nutrients, like minerals, creating empty spaces in which circulating foreign materials like toxic metals and chemicals accumulate. Each mineral in the body is associated with an emotional issue and, thus, nutrient deficiencies or imbalances from adrenal fatigue or adrenal burnout always affect the individual emotionally in varying degrees.

For instance, there are three degrees of anxiety: situational anxiety, general anxiety, and panic attacks. There are also three degrees of depression: situational depression, clinical depression, and major depression. The body's ability to maintain homeostasis, or to recover through adequate nutrition, prevents the individual from moving into the second and third degrees of these emotional states.

Magnesium promotes relaxation. Zinc supports stability; chromium prompts flexibility. Calcium is protective; potassium provides adaptive energy; and sodium responds for emergency energy. In their balanced state, each of these minerals increases homeostasis, leading to calming or anti-aggressive and anti-violent responses.

These particular minerals are also base (alkaline) and necessary to balance pH levels in the body. If these important alkaline minerals are deficient, then acid will increase and cause inflammation. Inflammation can affect any part of the body—digestive tract (leaky gut syndrome), joints, muscles, brain, etc. These calming nutrients and other amino acids are necessary for proper neurotransmitter function in the brain. Persons who are deficient in these nutrients will be depressed, anxious, and unable to sleep well and experience other gut-brain associated issues.

As these minerals are depleted day after day and month after month through a poor diet, stress, and other factors, the individual becomes less resilient to life's challenges and relies on addictive substances and behaviors. In addition to sugar, addictive substances such as caffeine, drugs (prescription or recreational), tobacco, and alcohol are immediate fixes for the depressed person in adrenal burnout.

Chemicals from these substances provide a temporary high from the low physical and emotional states but are dangerous in the long run. All of the above symptoms are related to a severe energy deficit, and many of these behaviors represent various adaptations to that depletion. That is, the person is compensating for lack of energy by changing behavior. An individual may be attracted to various stimulants and drugs to relieve depression and provide a sense of feeling alive and well, albeit temporarily.

Post-traumatic-stress-disorder (PTSD) is a good example of someone in need of adrenal support.

Many individuals with PTSD—as well as individuals with adrenal burnout not caused by severe trauma—try to fill the God-shaped need by turning to drugs and alcohol. Post-traumatic-stress-disorder (PTSD) is a good example of someone in need of adrenal support. Researchers who recognized the "fight-or-flight" response also recognized the "freeze-and-dissociate" response. Anyone who has been in adrenal burnout or has experienced PTSD readily understands what it means to freeze-and-dissociate. Sexual abuse survivors almost always refer to "going to a safe place" during the episode, especially after more than one occurrence.

The American Association for Marriage and Family Therapy identifies three types of PTSD:

1. **Acute**: when the symptoms last between one and three months after the trauma.

2. **Chronic:** when the symptoms last for a minimum of three months following the trauma.

3. **Delayed**: when symptoms do not manifest for at least six months after the trauma. This is often found with adult survivors of childhood traumas.

Sexual abuse, incest, physical and emotional abuse, religious abuse, military combat, torture, severe childhood neglect, witnessing or being involved in a terrifying or life-threatening incident, and homicide or accident survival, occurring at any age are typical kinds of PTSD. PTSD can be triggered when the individual re-experiences intense fear creating severe anxiety, flashbacks, uncontrollable thoughts, and nightmares. These are common symptoms and can become chronic if help is not received.

These models of physical or emotional pain and suffering require adrenal investigation and renewal.

The Competition of Copper and Zinc

Adrenal stress creates continued miscommunication between the brain and gut and plays a huge role in digestion and the diagnosis of IBS (Irritable Bowel Syndrome) and IBD (Inflammatory Bowel Disease). Persons in adrenal burnout almost always have digestive problems such as gas, bloating, belching, heartburn, or gastric reflux. As they move from adrenal fatigue toward adrenal burnout, hydrochloric acid production in the stomach diminishes their ability to adequately digest animal protein diminishes accordingly. A feeling of heaviness in the stomach and general fatigue after eating meat protein are common for those suffering from adrenal burnout. Consequently, many in adrenal burnout avoid meat. To their further detriment, many become vegans consuming very little protein and denying themselves critical amino acids that would actually rebuild the adrenals.

The inability to digest meat can be further compromised by elevated copper as shown on a hair mineral analysis. A toxic copper level normally results from the inability to use copper especially if zinc level is also low. This usually means that copper will sequester, or bind itself up in the body, usually the liver. Copper toxicity will almost always cause a zinc deficiency because of their antagonistic relationship. Low zinc levels prevent the cells from utilizing glucose to absorb the necessary nutrition from the foods we eat to create energy. Zinc is also an important mineral for good immune function.

Copper is essential for energy production and to reduce excessive adrenal hormone activity. Deficient copper, whether bound up in tissue or frankly deficient, can be implicated in adrenal burnout. People in burnout sometimes suffer from an inability to use copper properly. Ceruloplasmin is a protein made in the liver that binds to copper, stores, and transports it to where it is needed, then releases it. Weakened adrenals cannot stimulate ceruloplasmin from the liver. When this happens, copper becomes biounavailable, compounding fatigue and simultaneously depleting zinc. In some cases, prolonged adrenal fatigue can lead to Wilson's disease, a disorder in which copper accumulates in the brain and liver.

Copper toxicity and zinc deficiency also interfere with pancreas' ability to secrete trypsin and chymotrypsin. These enzymes are required to digest meat protein. For the person in adrenal burnout who is also deficient in hydrochloric acid, digestion becomes a major difficulty resulting in gas, bloating, reflux, nausea, constipation, or diarrhea. As the condition progresses, poultry and fish become challenging to digest, too. For relief, the individual may turn to a totally vegetarian diet. The extent to which a person avoids meat protein provides a good subjective criterion for measuring adrenal insufficiency.

How to Identify Adrenal Cortisol Insufficiencies

Identifying whether you are suffering from adrenal fatigue or burnout can be performed in several ways. Please refer to previous pages to see if your body is manifesting the symptoms. In addition to these symptoms, an objective assessment of burnout can be made through mineral analysis of your hair or saliva testing. Hair analysis reveals the levels of minerals in the tissue of the body. With knowledge of these levels, especially sodium and potassium, we can ascertain the function of the adrenal glands and other organs and systems of the body and determine whether the person has adrenal fatigue or burnout. Hair analysis is also a great tool to identify copper's bioavailability or toxic buildup. Saliva testing identifies the cortisol levels four times throughout the day. This is a very good way to assess adrenal rhythm. Failure to address adrenal insufficiencies will impede healing in other areas.

Candace's Story of Recovery

Candace was five feet tall, weighing 115 pounds and 34 years old when I first saw her in 2006. Additionally, she experienced sinus infections at least five or six times a year for which she received antibiotics and steroids from her physician. She also suffered from painful digestive issues typically associated with ulcerative colitis.

During her first year under my care, we methodically addressed test results indicating adrenal burnout with elevated copper, found in hair analysis, low DHEA, and low Vitamin D levels. Dietary and other deficient nutrition levels were addressed, along with other therapies such as liver-gallbladder flush, deep diaphragmatic breathing, and dry skin brushing. Within a year Candace was completely off the colitis medication and no longer suffered from sinusitis or digestive issues.

She continues to check in with me and to improve and stabilize. At age 42, she gave birth to her first child (a beautiful baby girl), and two years later gave birth to precious twin boys. Her most recent colonoscopy showed no active colitis and no polyps.

Physical, Spiritual, & Emotional Recovery from Burnout

Those who have not suffered from adrenal burnout might easily say, "buck up, pull yourself up by the bootstraps, and get over it." But for those who are severely exhausted, this kind of willpower is elusive.

Recovery from burnout is a complex task, which cannot be rushed and must be accomplished gently and in stages. Changes should be made to lifestyle and diet, but spiritual implications should not be ignored in the recovery process. Your physical, emotional, and spiritual health are intertwined and function in tandem with body, soul, and spirit.

Stress almost always involves fear; the antidote to fear is always faith.

Reducing known stressors where you can, and changing your attitude toward those outside your control are critical. Fear of failure, not having enough, sickness and pain, rejection or abandonment, or being unsafe are all stressful. Many of these relate to spiritual bondages from as far back as when you were in the womb. Stress almost always involves fear; the antidote to fear is always faith, not of itself, but in whom it is placed. To have faith, you must believe and trust in what or whom your faith is placed. That Person is the one, true God, who will do what He has promised. Know Him by reading His revealed truth in the Bible. If you ask Him and trust Him, He will wipe away all your fears. Your life may not be perfect, but He has a plan for your perfection.

Restoring adrenal health requires quiet times of reflection and meditation. Begin journaling by making a list of stressors in your life. Eliminate those things that don't line up with who God created you to be and your goal of recovery. Of those that remain, reduce or delegate the least important ones. Make another list and write down what is most important in your life. Identify your purpose. Eliminate those things or relationships that don't line up with who you are and what is most important to you.

You cannot make lifestyle changes if you do not consider yourself important or worthy. As you become more spiritually healthy and realize how much you matter to God our Father through His unconditional love, it becomes easier to make adjustments. Recreate your attitude by acknowledging that operating the world is not your responsibility. The world is God's responsibility, and He is in control. Your responsibility is to listen, obey, and be still and know that He is God (Psalm 46:10). Allow God to change and restore you through His great mercy and grace.

Adrenal recovery involves taking the necessary time for rest and sleep. Take a thirty-minute nap each afternoon, if you are able. If night-time sleep is difficult for you, take time to relax before bed, close all electronic equipment, and take a bath in Epsom salts with lavender one hour before bed. Ten deep diaphragmatic breaths are very helpful, as well. The enemy wants to rob you of regenerative and restorative sleep. Meditating on God's Word before bed is always a good idea.

The enemy wants to rob you of regenerative and restorative sleep.

Dietary Changes: When Willpower Isn't Enough

Changing dietary intake is a crucial step in recovery from adrenal burnout. A person with inadequate energy reserve will be unable to stick to the typical low-calorie diet. The "yo-yo" diet syndrome and other common dieting disorders in our society often result in burnout. Some of these include a very low fat diet, vegetarianism, sugar addiction, and appetite disorders such as anorexia and bulimia.

During the re-entry phases to normal adrenal function, sugar cravings are not uncommon. Sugar craving resulting from inadequate adrenal response may be a necessary defense to avoid an impending catastrophe. The brain lacks the ability to store sugar, and if blood sugar (glucose) levels drop below about 50 mg/100 ml, an individual will frequently experience anxiety or panic attacks, behavioral disorders, drug or alcohol addiction, or violent or suicidal thoughts. Because sugar is the simplest form of fuel, the body can use and burn it for energy exactly as it is without drawing energy from an already depleted digestive system.

Withdrawal headaches are also common for the first day or two. Blood sugar regulation depends upon many factors, including optimal adrenal activity, the insulin secretion, optimal liver function, and adequate digestion and assimilation of carbohydrates and fats. The best way to eliminate these headaches is to keep blood sugar balanced by eating a few bites of protein and fat every two to

Including a nutrient dense breakfast is critical to restoring adrenal function.

three hours. This will also help prevent sugar cravings.

Including a nutrient-dense breakfast is critical to restoring adrenal function. Choose one that contains twenty to thirty grams of protein, an essential fatty acid such as coconut oil or flax meal, and a complex carbohydrate fruit or vegetable. A perfect restoration breakfast is a pea or rice protein shake with two tablespoons ground flaxseed and a fruit/veggie. Blended together with water and almond or coconut milk, this combination is more easily digested than a whole protein such as eggs.

The fat and protein help to balance blood sugar level longer. Eating five or six smaller meals throughout the day for a while will increase your metabolic rate and prevent further breakdown of lean muscle mass. Concentrate on chewing each mouthful well to lessen the digestive burden. Contrary to popular bias against eating close to bedtime, if you suffer from adrenal burnout, you will contribute to your recovery by having a few bites of protein and fat an hour or so before bed. This will prevent blood sugar dips and provide restorative sleep.

The kind of exercise that you do while in adrenal recovery is very important, too. In fact, many people drive themselves into adrenal burnout by over-exercising. Moderate exercise will support recovery and might include yoga, Pilates, walking, and light weight lifting. Strenuous aerobic exercise such as running or competitive sports is not recommended because your adrenals cannot respond to the resultant demand for additional hormones which will interfere with recovery. Determining you body's baseline fat and lean percentages is important to ensure that you are increasing—and not breaking down—lean muscle mass as you recover.

Eating, exercising, resting, and meditating as recommended, as well as drinking one-half ounce of purified water for each pound that you weigh will ensure adrenal recovery and weight loss in the form of fat and not lean muscle tissue.

Nutrients for Adrenal Recovery

Choosing health supplements for any health issue, but especially adrenal recovery, can be tricky and confusing to accomplish on your own. You should enlist the support of a qualified health care professional to identify other areas of involvement other than the adrenal glands, such as digestion, thyroid, liver, gallbladder, lymph, lungs, colon, etc.

For more complete health restoration, refer to the chapters in this book on detoxification and release of heavy metals, chemicals, parasites, fungus, bacteria, and virus. However, do not undertake this until you are at least three weeks into adrenal recovery. While these toxins burden the body, the adrenals need to be able to carry out their part in the detoxification process, too.

Supplements such as Vitamins A, B, C, D, and E and minerals such as magnesium, calcium, zinc, manganese, or copper, and other glandulars should be a focus of any supplement protocol for adrenal recovery. Vitamins are required for the chemical reactions that produce energy. For example, the B-complex vitamins are required in the energy cycles, where final conversion of food to energy takes place in each body cell. As with minerals, an optimum amount of each vitamin is required. Excessive amounts of vitamins over extended periods of time, especially the oil-soluble A, D, E, and K, can cause health problems. See more about nutrients in Part Six, Rebuilding with Micronutrient Supplementation.

Restore digestion by incorporating the right foods and adding soothing digestive substances, hydrochloric acid, and other enzymes. A high-quality, multi-strain probiotic will also help to support digestion, absorption, and elimination. An amino acid like l-glutamine will help to heal the gut and is especially beneficial for relief from sugar cravings. Remember that you may need only a small supplemental regimen at first depending on your state of health.

Rhodiola rosea reduces fatigue, improves mental focus and concentration, and relieves anxiety. Low doses (100 mg) taken one-three times daily are effective for fatigue, while much higher doses (300-600 mg) taken one-three times daily work well if you are suffering from anxiety, too.

Phosphatidylserine (PS) protects against dysregulation of the HPA (hypothalamic-pituitary-adrenal) axis that occurs after chronic stress.

Theanine is a simple amino acid that has been researched for stress and anxiety and can be taken in 100-200 mg doses one-three times throughout the day and before bed.

Vitamin C and other antioxidants are effective anti-inflammatories. Since vitamin C is not stored in the body (except for a small portion of the adrenal glands), it should be taken throughout the day in approximately 600 mg doses, three-four times per day.

Ginsengs are among the class of herbs known as adaptogens and are very good for stabilizing cortisol levels for someone in adrenal fatigue.

Omega 3 essential fatty acids have been studied for stress-buffering anti-inflammatory effects.

Adrenal glandular extracts are recommended for adrenal burnout only and for no longer than one-three months depending on your overall health.

From Hopeless to Fantastic

Thirty-eight-year-old Michael (not his real name) was diagnosed ten years prior with bipolar (manic-depressive) disorder. On his first visit to my office, he revealed that he was in a depressive state for the past three and one-half years, could not work, and had gained over fifty pounds. He disclosed that "over the years I have been on numerous, too many to recall, prescription medications, with many side effects, and nothing ever worked for me." He admitted contemplating suicide, and that being in my office was his last hope.

I started him on the recommended protocol and within two weeks he noticed a change. Over the course of the next few months, he discontinued most of the bipolar meds and eliminated Adderall for adult ADD under his physician's supervision. He reported, "I am starting to come out of my depression and feel positive improvements in my whole life for the first time in four years."

He now has lost approximately forty-five pounds and says he feels fantastic! He says, "This has been a life-changing event for me. I was ready to give up just a few short months ago, but something led me to Nutritional Direction to get the help and guidance I needed. Without that support, I do not know where I would be today."

Part Five

The Role of Inflammation in Depression and Anxiety

Inflammation

Should it surprise anyone that the immune system is compromised during times of stress and that illnesses increase and even become chronic? Many studies, such as one by the Carnegie Melon Institute in Pittsburgh, have confirmed the relationship between stress and illness. These illnesses are not limited to colds and flu but expand into asthma, allergies, chronic respiratory infections, arthritis, and other autoimmune diseases, which lay a tragic foundation for more debilitating diseases like Lupus, CFIDS (chronic fatigue immune dysfunction syndrome), fibromyalgia, rheumatoid arthritis, and others.

Dr. DicQie Fuller-Looney, Ph.D., DrSc, ND, CNC, a trail-blazer in enzyme research and clinical application, and founder of *Transformation Enzyme Corporation* in Houston, states that:

> "Health Science now links many diseases or disorders under one flagship heading called Neuro-Immune Dysfunction Syndrome (NIDS). The second brain in the gut communicates through the central nervous system with the primary brain in the cranial cavity. When stress activates the flight or fight response in the central nervous system, digestion can shut down because your central nervous system shuts down blood flow, affecting the contraction of your digestive muscles and decreasing secretions needed for digestion. Stress can also cause inflammation of the gut, making you more susceptible to infection."

Other research shows that the effects of psychological stress impair the body's ability to regulate inflammation and can promote the development and progression of disease. Cohen and his research colleagues found that "Because inflammation plays an important role in the onset and progression of a wide range of diseases, this model may have broad implications for understanding the role of stress in health."

Inflammation is a critical piece of the puzzle to overcome anxiety, depression, and fatigue. These illnesses could be referred

... identifying the root cause is key to unlocking long-term health.

to as a "silent" inflammation of the brain. If you've ever seen someone with the "loud" inflammatory pain of arthritis, or have experienced a severe muscle strain or tendonitis, you understand the inflammation your brain is experiencing with overactive immune stimulation.

Some professionals believe that inflammation is the root of all disease. I respectfully disagree for two reasons. The first is that some inflammation is healthy, such as the inflammatory process that heals wounds either an unintentionally inflicted cut, or intentionally inflicted such as rotator cuff surgery. Inflammation is necessary to heal a cut or a cold. Secondly, inflammation is an invaluable signal of an unhealthy underlying condition. In other words, we have to go deeper to find the root of inflammation itself.

In pathophysiology as discussed throughout this book, identifying the root cause is key to unlocking long-term health. Clearly, alleviating anxiety, depression, and fatigue begins at a deeper root than inflammation. You can see from the following hypothesis that inflammation is process number five.

1. Gluten and other questionable foods produce a destructive protein called zonulin.
2. Zonulin and dysregulation in the HPA axis and the gut-brain axis cause leaky gut.
3. Leaky gut triggers immune system response.
4. Immune system releases chemicals called cytokines.
5. Pro-inflammatory cytokines generate inflammation.
6. Poor adrenal cortisol function cannot regulate inflammatory response.
7. Unregulated and prolonged inflammation and imbalanced gut microbiome influence mental issues.
8. Mental issues, in turn, exacerbate intestinal symptoms.

A plethora of research, including a study published in the Journal of Neuroinflammation in September 2014, shows that leaky gut can cause various neurocognitive disorders. For example, intestinal permeability (leaky gut) triggers the immune system to release pro-inflammatory cytokines and other chemicals implicated in depression. Cytokines are chemical messengers produced by the immune system much the same as neurotransmitters are chemical messengers of the central nervous system and hormones are chemical messengers of the endocrine system. Cytokines such as IL-l, IL-6 and TNF-alpha are produced to fight infections from any number of invaders or pathogens that the body recognizes as unfriendly, including foods. They are also produced in response to sleep deprivation or other stressful issues and elevation of cortisol by the adrenal glands.

Cytokines are not a bad thing. They are critical to healing in appropriate doses. However, they become destructive when produced in excess and over prolonged periods, much the same as cortisol or insulin. In excessive amounts, they alter enzyme response, thereby depleting serotonin and driving up quinolinic acid and causing brain inflammation. Research has also shown that the clostridia bacteria produces metabolites that inhibit the dopamine-beta-hydroxylase enzyme which converts dopamine to norepinephrine. These neurotransmitters are influential in mental disorders ranging from anxiety, panic attacks, depression, Parkinson's, and Alzheimer's. Lipopolysaccharide (LPS) produced by a leaky gut also stimulate cytokine response driving anxiety and depression. Asthma and allergies are also driven by the pro-inflammatory response of the immune system. As such, the immune system is a critical regulator in the inflammatory model of these disorders.

Additionally, prolonged periods of stress alter cortisol's effectiveness to down-regulate the inflammatory response because the tissue sensitivity to the hormone is decreased. For a dispensed hormone to be effective, it must also be received by a healthy tissue receptor. Thus, poor gut function can also be implicated in hormonal deficiencies and imbalances. "Inflammation is partly regulated by the hormone cortisol, and when cortisol is not allowed to serve this function, inflammation can get out of control," said Cohen, Professor of Psychology at Dietrich College of Humanities and Social Sciences.

The tight junctions of the small and large intestines, supported by mucosal tissue, create a protective barrier from the rest of the body. In 2000, Dr. Alessio Fasano and his team at the University of Maryland's School of Medicine discovered a protein called zonulin. This destructive protein, when produced in excess by ingesting foods such as gluten, instigates breakdown of the mucosal cells and causes these tight junction barriers to loosen and allow microscopic molecules to escape the intestinal tract through the "leaky gut."

The immune system, then, properly responds by releasing pro-inflammatory cytokines which in turn may lead to the development of depressive symptoms, often coupled with anxiety, bipolar disorder, or schizophrenia. Without the proper support of the adrenal glands secretion of cortisol and other hormones, this problem will be exacerbated. Microbial infections can further burden these mental issues since the immune system responds, in the same way, issuing regulatory and pro-inflammatory cytokines leading to inflammation and causing depression and anxiety.

These pro-inflammatory cytokines cause further loosening of the tight junctions of the gut. The probiotic strain and species Bifidobacterium breve have the ability to down-regulate these pro-inflammatory cytokines. Vitamin D is also an excellent modulator of inflammation directly through cell trafficking in the immune system. Due to Vitamin D's anti-inflammatory capability, it can prevent a wide range of inflammatory diseases including intestinal bowel diseases, depression, colon cancer, and hormone-related breast, prostate, uterine, and ovarian cancer.

These pro-inflammatory cytokines cause further loosening of the tight junctions of the gut.

The Gut-Brain Axis: A Breakthrough for Hope

We have previously discussed the importance of the hypothalamic-pituitary-adrenal (HPA) axis as a critical governor of stress. Dysregulation in this axis compromises the adrenals and can also result in abdominal pain, inflammation, and intestinal permeability (leaky gut) leading to depression, schizophrenia, and anxiety. Studies have also shown that these mental issues can, in turn, worsen intestinal symptoms. Not only is the HPA axis crucial as it interacts with the gut-brain axis, but the entire microbiome of the gut is a key regulator of many of these same neuropsychiatric illnesses.

The science of Neurogastroenterology actually identifies a second brain in the bowel. Dr. Michael D. Gershon, M.D., author of "The Second Brain" published in 1998, calls rediscovery of the brain in the bowel a breakthrough for hope. The gut-brain axis uses the pathways of nerve transmission, hormones, and the immune system to communicate, so the axis can also be referred to as the Gastroneuro-endoimmune system.

This second brain, which is a part of the enteric nervous system embedded in the lining of the gastrointestinal tract, includes an element of the central nervous system. The second brain is not the seat of conscious thought or decision making, but, through rapid neuronal signaling, can greatly enhance or seriously interfere with the proper function of the gastrointestinal system. Microorganisms in the gut manufacture serotonin and GABA and operate through this gut-brain axis. The vagus nerve provides this two-way communication between the brain and the gut. For every one nerve fiber firing messages from the brain to the gut, nine others return information from the gut to the brain.

The central nervous system can influence peristaltic action (intestinal contractions that move the contents forward), sensation, secretion, inflammation, and gut disturbance. In turn, those processes influence mental and emotional status. These independent

Trying to digest food properly while under stress is not physiologically possible.

functions and reflexes support the autonomic nervous system, which does not require conscious thought.

If you have ever felt butterflies in your stomach before giving a speech, lost your appetite upon meeting a new boy/girlfriend, had a "gut feeling", or faced intestinal urgency (diarrhea) the night before an examination, then you have personally experienced the actions of the dual nervous systems and the brain-gut connection.

Trying to digest food properly while under stress is not physiologically possible. As we have already seen in discussions on adrenal function, the body diverts blood from the digestive system to fuel the brain and other parts of the body when we are under stress. Low hydrochloric acid production in the stomach is very bad news for a stressed body, especially when trying to dismantle and kill E.coli and other pathogenic foodborne bacteria. In 1923, the French scientist, Dr. H. Baruk, discovered that the E.coli bacteria, when permitted residence in the human gastrointestinal tract, produces a toxin that can cause nervous system disorders such as schizophrenia. In much the same way, other bacteria in the gut manufacture chemicals that change brain signaling, which can cause anxiety, depression, cravings, addictions, and insomnia.

Recognizing that God created you to work as a whole being—spirit, soul, and body—as the gut-brain axis demonstrates, provides a breakthrough for hope. Not a single system or part of your being can be divorced from the others. They support one another synergistically in the body's on-going, God-designed process to heal itself. Getting to the root cause can take time. But identifying the root cause removes the burden from those over-worked systems and, through nutritional therapies, allows them to return to normal function.

This model of disease process for anxiety, depression, and fatigue also gives hope to the individual suffering. The research also persuades against applying a bandage antidepressant or anti-anxiety prescription without uncovering the real cause of these psychological symptoms. In 2008, Turner and associates published a study in which they reviewed all literature and data reported by the FDA concerning the benefits of antidepressants. They discovered that a full one-half of antidepressant trials failed to show any benefit over a placebo. These scientists found that study results were only reported for primarily positive outcomes.

Not a single system or part of your being can be divorced from the others. They support one another synergistically in the body's on-going, God-designed process to heal itself.

A Clinical Testimony for Root-Cause Analogy

Several years ago I counseled with a thirty-two-year-old woman with profound anxiety. Her test results for gluten sensitivity were higher than laboratory test parameters could measure... in other words, off the charts. I have never seen higher test results. She agreed to a gluten-, dairy-, and sugar-free diet until her two-week follow-up appointment. In ten days she called me to report that she had experienced no anxiety for the previous three days. "How is that possible?" she asked.

Thyroid Inflammation

Discussing the role inflammation plays in depression, anxiety, and fatigue would be incomplete without addressing the thyroid gland.This gland incorporates the parathyroid gland and surrounds the Adam's apple. It has many responsibilities, not the least of which is to stabilize metabolism and energy. The thyroid glands, along with the adrenals, are responsible for almost 90% of metabolic activity. Dysregulation of either of these glands can easily lead to depression, anxiety, fatigue, weight gain, impaired cellular energy

The thyroid glands, along with the adrenals, are responsible for almost 90% of metabolic activity.

regulation, and many other concerns. Like the adrenal glands, the thyroid gland is controlled by the hypothalamus and pituitary glands in the cranial cavity, so its message pathway is referred to as the HPT axis.

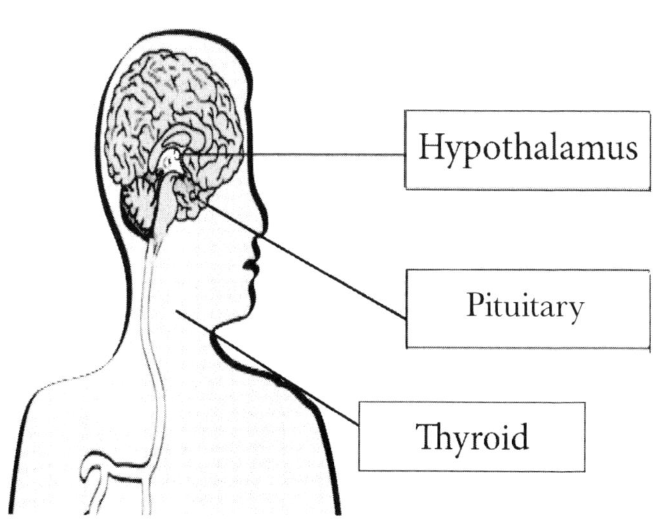

Upon receiving informational hormones from the hypothalamus and pituitary glands, the thyroid produces an enzyme called thyroid peroxidase (TPO). This enzyme combines with hydrogen peroxide and iodine to create T4 and T3 hormones. Thyroid stimulating hormone (TSH) from the pituitary signals the thyroid gland to produce a protein called thyroglobulin. This protein combines with iodine to produce more T4, which is released into the bloodstream. The liver then converts T4 to T3 through the glucuronidation and sulfation pathways. These are pathways, like the methylation pathway discussed earlier, that carry out jobs uniquely their own.

The healthy intestinal tract also converts about twenty percent of T4 into T3. Without a well-functioning liver and a well-balanced gut microbiome the extra twenty percent might be lost.

Hashimoto's thyroiditis is an autoimmune and inflammatory disease directed at the thyroid hormones. This disease most often causes hypo (low) thyroid function, but can also cause the thyroid to operate in overdrive, depending on the health of the gut, adrenals, and other organs or glands. The immune system misinterprets the thyroid hormones as foreign invaders and disengages them before their receptor site can absorb them, essentially negating the initial production. Standard blood tests are inconclusive to reveal the malfunction because they only measure the level of the produced hormone, not what the receptor site received to complete the message cycle. The Hashimoto's blood test is more conclusive because it measures the antibodies that the immune system created to disengage the thyroid hormones.

The antibodies reveal the extent of inflammation and a dysregulated immune system. The thyroid hormones are disengaged or rendered powerless and taken out of action. Some describe this as the immune system attacking the thyroid hormones. While this may be true, it makes the immune system look like the bad guy, when in fact, going back to the root cause and finding the real "bad guy" should be our mindset. The specific hormone receptor antibodies produced by the immune system target thyroid peroxidase and thyroglobulin enzymes. If both of these enzyme antibodies are elevated in blood work, the resultant diagnosis would be autoimmune thyroiditis, also known as Hashimoto's disease. Much research has shown that hypothyroidism and Hashimoto's can be directly related to depression and anxiety, especially in conjunction with an adrenal system that is not working properly.

Part Six

Restoring Mental and Emotional Health through the Gut Highway

Detoxification to Prevent Foundational Stages of Disease

Corrie ten Boom was a Dutch Christian whose family helped hide and plan escape routes for Jews during World War II and the Nazi Holocaust. I love what her father said to her as he insisted on carrying her suitcase to the train, "Some knowledge is too heavy… you cannot bear it … your Father will carry it until you are able."

Like Corrie ten Boom, when I started on my personal road to reclaim my health, the little bit of information I had about toxic waste and detoxification could have been dangerous without the support of some wise health advisors. For instance, I had no idea that my magnesium stores were severely depleted and the critical role magnesium plays, being necessary for almost every metabolic process of the body. To force the body to cleanse and detoxify in the absence of vital nutrients can be dangerous. I am grateful for those individuals at that time, and I encourage you to find a trustworthy, qualified health care professional to support your road to recovery.

Allow me to differentiate between the terms "cleansing" and "detoxification." Cleansing generally refers to flushing out loose waste material, most often from the large bowel (colon). This can be accomplished in a couple of days. Detoxification, however, is a complete supplemental nutritional protocol that lasts anywhere from ten to thirty days (longer for those with more serious chronic issues). Detoxification and cleansing are generally accomplished simultaneously. The goal is to upregulate or optimize body systems that are regularly involved in these natural processes.

Like the cardiovascular, respiratory, and nervous systems, the body has a natural detoxification system. According to physician, Dr. Sherry A. Rogers, in her book, *Tired or Toxic*, traditional physicians do not study detoxification as a body system or one that can instigate healing. For conditions such as IBD (Inflammatory Bowel Disease), physicians are taught to address the symptoms with prednisone or anti-inflammatory drugs or by cutting out the inflamed portion of the intestine.

God created your body to detoxify naturally and continuously.

God created your body to detoxify naturally and continuously. Your body has three options to rid itself of toxins either ingested through food, water, your environment, or negative emotions, or created by imbalances or deficiencies in the body.

First Option: If the body is healthy and functioning properly, it will break down the toxin to make it less harmful and avoid damaging an exit pathway as it expels the toxin.

Second Option: If the cellular systems responsible for detoxifying and clearing are not working properly, then the toxin will be sent through the body unchanged, potentially wreaking havoc along the way.

Third Option: If the first and second options fail, then the body can store the harmful pollutant in the cellular structure indefinitely, initiating the foundational stages of disease.

The body heals in reverse chronological order. So it heals the cold you had last week before it heals the mononucleosis you had in college and before it heals the pneumonia you had as a child. It also heals from the inside out. A leaky gut heals before the final healing stages of a skin disorder. Healing the physical body will accelerate with spiritual healing and recovery by the Holy Spirit, who gives hope because of our faith in Him as the Healer.

Everyone can benefit from some form of cleansing or detoxification. Such a program will alleviate many common acute and chronic illnesses. The following is a short list of symptoms that indicate the body is burdened with toxic material and cleansing or detoxification would be beneficial:

- Digestive complaints of any kind
- Depression

- Anxiety and panic attacks
- Fatigue or lethargy
- Arthritis and other auto-immune illnesses
- Body odor or bad breath
- Insomnia
- Headaches
- Low back pain
- Poor memory or concentration
- Sciatica
- Asthma and allergies
- Chronic colds, flu and bronchitis
- Any disease

Periodic detoxification is important for an optimally functioning body and one of the best proactive steps you can take to expedite balanced physical and mental health. Trees are no better than their root system, and so it is with your body—you are no healthier than your "root system," the terrain of your gut.

> *For he will be like a tree planted by the water that extends its roots by a stream, and* ***will not fear*** *when the heat comes, but its leaves will be green, and it* ***will not be anxious*** *in a year of drought nor cease to yield fruit (emphasis mine).*
>
> Jeremiah 17:8

Cleansing, as previously mentioned, refers to clearing toxins and other potentially harmful debris from the body. The job of detoxifying, though, is shared among every organ and system of the body. The colon, liver, heart, lymphatic system, kidneys, respiratory system, skin, and even the immune system has a different role in detoxification and, at the same time, clearing the body of waste. Metabolic pathways become congested and overburdened with toxins and mucus or are otherwise unable to perform their jobs. Detoxification and cleansing support these

I like to describe these free radicals as live, on-fire wires in the body in search of "firefighter" nutrients to douse the fire.

pathways to enable the body to work at its optimum state to neutralize or transform toxins, clearing them along with excess mucus and congestion.

The body's thousands of metabolic processes generate free radicals. These are inflammatory molecules that cause oxidative stress and require antioxidants like vitamins A, C, D, and E and the minerals zinc and selenium, to deactivate them. I like to describe these free radicals as live, on-fire wires in the body in search of "firefighter" nutrients to douse the fire. Current research shows that oxidative stress is elevated and "firefighter" antioxidants are depleted in depressed and anxious individuals

Even exercise creates free radicals. Do you ever wonder why, when you embark on an exercise program after months or years of a sedentary lifestyle, you suddenly get sick? Repetitive large muscle movement releases stored toxins from the cellular structure. In the presence of an already weakened immune system, cold and flu-like symptoms will occur. The same thing can happen when you begin a detoxification program with a weakened immune system.

Exit Pathway Clearance

While system detoxification is important, removing the trash from the process is critical. Disposal is accomplished by ensuring that exit pathways are open and ready to clear. The colon and respiratory system, including eyes, ears, nose, and mouth, lymphatic system, kidneys, and skin are the exit pathways intended for clearing. If the skin is functioning as God designed, it should be able to eliminate even more waste than the colon. If the exit pathways are blocked, the body will recirculate the trash, and the intended cleansing process will cause further harm.

The detoxification process should also ensure that the organs and systems involved are supported with proper macro and micro nutrition. Comprehensive cleansing and detoxification formulas are available through qualified health care professionals.

Techniques for opening these pathways include:

- Skin—daily dry skin brushing with a natural bristle body brush prior to a shower, and zinc and vitamin C supplements

- Lymphatic system—natural herbals such as Echinacea and jumping on a trampoline

- Colon—vitamin C, buffered with minerals to prevent intestinal discomfort, until loose stool forms (bowel tolerance) or magnesium citrate to bowel tolerance

- Kidneys—natural herbals such as uva-ursi, hydrangea, marshmallow root, or parsley

- Respiratory—herbals such as eucalyptus, oregano, lobelia, fenugreek, and mullein

Detoxification must take place in steps to prevent becoming even sicker than you were when you started. Even if you feel healthy, toxins deposited at the cellular level may not yet have triggered symptoms, you might still become sick during the initial steps. Use the following as a guideline:

1. Support the immune system with immune-enhancing supplements.

2. Be sure the lymph and colon are up-regulated to function properly.

3. Confirm that other exit pathways such as the skin, kidneys, and respiratory system are open and clearing properly.

4. Change your dietary intake to remove harmful or interference foods. (More information can be found in *"Dietary Changes for Recovery and Locked-In Healing" later in Part Six*).

5. Add support for liver and gallbladder detoxification.

6. Kill and rid the body of yeast and fungus, virus, bacteria, parasites, heavy metals, and chemicals.

For very sick individuals—especially those experiencing chronic symptoms or diagnosed with serious health issues—the detoxification process should take months to accomplish. Those who just want to improve good health and want to rid themselves of pesky symptoms could combine Steps 1 through 4 for one week, then add Step 5 in the second week. Then in the third week, combine Step 6 with Steps 4 and 5. Steps 1, 2, and 3 need only be continued if those pathways are having trouble staying open.

One and Done?

When referring to cleansing and detoxification, many people think about removing all the trash or toxic waste build-up in the body at one time. They imagine themselves spending the majority of their time in the bathroom and might also think, "one and done." However, accumulated waste material becomes toxic and hardened over the years. It can rigidly attach itself to the twenty-six-foot-long intestinal wall and may take many months to remove in a healthy manner.

Incidentally, many people mistakenly think that the diarrhea-causing bowel preparation used the night before a colonoscopy is an adequate cleanse, but the product itself actually introduces chemicals that are harmful to the body. These products, as well as many over-the-counter laxatives, contain polyethylene glycol manufactured by stringing together molecules of ethylene glycol into a large polymer chain—hence the prefix poly. Ethylene glycol, by itself, is used to manufacture automotive antifreeze and brake fluid. According to the National Institute for Occupational Safety and Health, it is an extremely toxic substance.

Ethylene glycol is chemically broken down in the body into toxic compounds. It and its toxic byproducts first affect the central nervous system (CNS), then the heart, and finally the kidneys. Ingestion of sufficient amounts, as little as 30 ml, can be fatal.

In 2011, the U.S. Food and Drug Administration issued an adverse event warning of "neuropsychiatric events" from ingesting polyethylene glycol products, such as Miralax, an over-the-counter laxative.

In addition to harmful build-up of accumulated debris the accumulation sometimes functions as a protective mechanism, binding to and becoming part of certain organs or systems. For instance, calcium might be re-assigned from bone to other tissue to protect against harmful heavy metals. In this way, redirected nutrients become depleted from their proper source and a functional disease such as osteoporosis begins.

Spiritual Roots that Impede Physical & Emotional Healing

We clean the outside of our bodies every day; cleansing the inside occasionally is important as well. Internal cleansing and supporting natural detoxification should be part of a total protocol to alleviate and eliminate the symptoms of anxiety, depression, debilitating fatigue, allowing the body to return to optimal function and homeostasis.

During the process of physical cleansing and detoxification, you will not only feel lighter and healthier; your emotional outlook will improve, too. You may be surprised to discover that your thoughts and emotions can overburden your body on a cellular level. Each thought and every emotion, whether negative or positive, has a biochemical response that must be metabolized by the body's detoxification organs and systems. Unresolved negative emotions of anger, bitterness, fear, rejection, and others can wound deeply, triggering formation of harmful chemical byproducts. If the byproducts are not expelled, then they are stored in the cellular tissue, creating soul sicknesses: anxiety, depression, and other psychological maladies.

Often these chemical byproducts become lodged in what is known as the acupuncture meridian system. This is another system of the body consisting of twelve major meridians (pathways that allow message and energy flow). Like the hormonal or central nervous systems, the acupuncture meridian system transfers energy messages throughout the body. Blocked energy flow created by toxic negative thoughts and emotional byproducts will result in some or all of the energy being cut off to that organ, interfering with health and vitality.

A simple example of this is an infection in the mouth or a dental cavity filled with a "silver" (toxic mercury) filling. All of the body's twelve major meridians travel through the teeth. Each tooth represents a particular meridian. For example, the kidney meridian runs through the two front teeth. The kidneys are responsible for regulating sodium and potassium levels to support healthy cardiovascular pressure.

In my practice, I use an electro-dermal screening machine, which assesses electrical interferences in the meridian pathways. Several years ago, a client who was evaluated on this machine showed to have an infection in those two front teeth. She experienced no pain. But I insisted that she seek treatment from a biological dentist (one who practices holistic dentistry and is well-informed about the meridian flow of energy through each tooth and its relationship with the health of the entire body). She finally agreed to go, and the dentist did, in fact, locate and clear an infection in those teeth. The woman's blood pressure immediately returned to normal, which is the reason she was seeing me—she wanted to get off her blood pressure medication. Any infection, heavy metal toxicity (which includes mercury), or any other focal disturbance that interferes with energy flow through these meridians will cause health problems.

Byproducts of negative emotions increase acid in the body.

Inflammation, as was addressed extensively in Part Five, is another example of how these energy blockages might occur. Byproducts of negative emotions increase acid in the body. The healthy body maintains a steady balance of acidity and alkalinity. When the balance becomes skewed toward acidity, inflammatory processes occur and disease begins at the cellular level. Where there's pain, there's inflammation. However, the reverse is not always true—inflammation will not always cause pain. Arteriosclerosis and continually elevated cortisol or insulin levels are painless examples of destructive inflammation—silent functional disease processes. Even cancer is a silent inflammatory disease in the early stages that impedes cellular communication.

He Peels, Reveals, and Heals

Cleansing and detoxification is an amazing picture of how the Heavenly Father peels, reveals, and heals, not only from a physiological perspective, but also on a mental and emotional level. Depression was one of the key issues that I struggled with during my physical and emotional crisis. Many years ago, as I was asking the Holy Spirit to help unravel my condition, I wrote in my journal:

> "I spend one-half my life in guilt, and the other half in shame, wondering what people will think about me sprinkled in the gaps. God has been showing me plenty about guilt and shame this last week—that it takes an

> extraordinary amount of pride to wallow in guilt and shame. That very pride interferes with my ability to forgive myself. Plus it negates the power of Jesus's shed blood on the cross for my sins! I may as well literally slap Him in the face... how arrogant I am! I need to lift up my head and look to Jesus Christ. Let me touch the hem of His garment and be healed!"

After I had written those sentences in my journal, I realized the Holy Spirit had revealed that the source of my depression at the spiritual level was guilt and shame. I had believed foundational lies about myself from the enemy since my childhood. By the age of sixteen (even though I did not recognize it at the time), the guilt and shame morphed into a spirit of condemnation and loathing for myself. By the age of thirty-nine, my physical body began to break down, due in large part to layer upon layer of spiritual bondage and oppression. My gut twisted with physical pain most days, and my brain sifted through intense fog every day. But one day as He was peeling back the layers of physical and emotional pain, God revealed to me that what I ate affected how I felt, not only physically, but emotionally, too.

During that time, while on a sales call with my boss, I suffered an attack of abdominal pain with nausea and profuse sweating in the client's office. I excused myself and proceeded to the restroom, desperately trying to walk upright. But the pain was too great. I remember wondering how cooked onions could cause that kind of pain. What I didn't know was the incredible burden of toxins—physically, emotionally, and spiritually—that I was carrying. Neither was I aware that I was in adrenal burnout. Plus, I had eaten lunch under stress, making digestion an extreme challenge for my already compromised body. That was my first clue how closely intertwined my diet was to my mental, emotional, and physical well-being.

Identifying and releasing spiritual bondages—a process of nourishing the soul—is the most important step in completely restoring health. One of the best ways to accomplish this is through the support of a Christian Licensed Professional Counselor (LPC) or Psychologist. Additionally, time spent interacting with Jesus Christ, the greatest Counselor and Healer, and journaling will help you travel the road to personal health. Addressing spiritual bondage always expedites simultaneous physical and emotional healing. He longs to show all things to you. Trust Him to peel back the layers of pain and toxins for you physically and emotionally, to reveal what He wants you to know, and to be healed according to His perfect timing.

Identifying and releasing spiritual bondages—a process of nourishing the soul—is the most important step in completely restoring health.

You are a spiritual being, in a physical body, with a soul. The soul consists of mind, will, and emotions and, thereby, thinks, makes choices, and feels. When natural detoxification processes are overburdened, the chemical byproducts of toxic thoughts and emotions are deposited in various organs, glands, and systems of the body. Left unchecked and allowed to fester, these can become forms of spiritual bondage. Cleansing, detoxification, and spiritual healing clear up congestion in these pathways, allowing electrical energy to flow once again unimpeded.

- Bitterness is stored in the gall bladder.
- Anger, frustration, jealousy, and envy are stored in the liver and gallbladder.
- Grief, hate, and impatience are stored in the heart and small intestine.
- Fear is stored in the respiratory system and kidneys.

- Worry, anxiety, and mistrust are stored in the stomach and pancreas.
- Sorrow is stored in the pancreas.
- Guilt, shame, and depression are stored in lungs, skin, and large intestine.

Anger is almost always a secondary emotion. The primary emotion might be fear, and the spiritual root of fear might be abandonment. The antidote to fear of any kind is always faith … not faith itself, but in the only One in whom you can ultimately place your trust—Jesus Christ. A Christian counselor can help identify the primary emotion or deeper spiritual root, which will expedite the body's response to healing protocols.

Many perfectionists, or people needing to be in control, suffer with colon and bowel problems. Controlling tendencies are often the outcome of feeling unprotected or unsafe, especially during a traumatic childhood event. Perfectionist tendencies often result from toxic guilt and shame about doing a "bad" thing (feelings which should belong to the perpetrator), or not being "good enough." Many times these individuals suffer from post-traumatic stress disorder (PTSD), an issue that always requires adrenal support.

Addressing revolving negative thoughts and emotions is indispensable in building a framework for making choices in harmony with God's original design for your body, spirit, and soul, and to allow you to hear His voice more clearly. 2 Corinthians 10:5 instructs us to take every thought captive. "We are destroying speculations, and every lofty thing raised up against the knowledge of God, and we are taking every thought captive to the obedience of Christ." Capture and trap those negative thoughts, wrap them in a psychological garbage bag like the trash they are, and destroy them. Cleansing, revitalizing, healing and regenerating your soul cannot be ignored in your quest for balanced and locked-in healing.

When you begin the detoxification process, you may re-experience repressed emotions within a few days, weeks, or months as toxins are released from storage, detoxified, and removed. How quickly these chemicals release depends on your level of toxic burden and how willing your body is to rid itself of toxins. During my many years of guiding clients through detoxification, the process had to be paused on quite a number of occasions because feelings of anger, bitterness, panic attacks, or severe clinical depression were too overwhelming to continue. Post-traumatic stress flashbacks and the process of releasing repressed emotions can be debilitating. My own experience taught me that forcing the body to continue in these cases is not a good idea. Stop the cleansing process, grab a journal, and begin asking and recording what it is that God wants to reveal to you. As He peels, He reveals and heals. This is an excellent opportunity to spend time building your relationship with Christ.

... grab a journal and begin asking and recording what it is that God wants to reveal to you.

Nutritional Therapy Has More Than One Benefit for Janice (not her real name)

"I began the program recommended by Dr. Price almost a month ago, and my quality of life has already drastically improved! I have spent the past eight years on and off antidepressants and even though they "took the edge off," I still didn't quite feel myself. I also had some of the negative side effects like weight gain that I struggled with. In the past month, my mood has been very stable, and my carbohydrate cravings have decreased, and I have finally begun losing some of my extra weight. I feel so much better knowing that I am actually replenishing deficiencies rather than just masking the feelings of depression with a drug that I do not know the long-term effects on my body. Nutritional Direction has been such a blessing!"

Restoring Digestive Function

Restoring the gastrointestinal tract—including digestion, absorption, and elimination—is perhaps the most critical step in any quest for health, with the exception of releasing spiritual bondages. The gastrointestinal tract, also known as the alimentary canal, is the body system that metabolizes, absorbs, and carries nutrients to support every single organ and cell of the body. Where would you get the nutrient precursors required for micro-processing in the brain, not to mention nutrients for natural detoxification, without the digestive process? Where would you get amino acids and essential fatty acids to stabilize blood sugar levels and prevent catabolism (breakdown) of lean muscle mass? Improper digestion and absorption can also upset the body's pH level, which is critical to life itself.

Proper digestive function can rarely be completely restored without embarking on an appropriately applied cleansing program. Many diseases, such as the inflammatory bowel diseases of ulcerative colitis, Crohn's disease, spastic colon, diverticulitis, and celiac sprue have an obvious connection to the gut and digestive function. However, diseases such as depression, anxiety, and fatigue are not so clearly connected to gut health. We've already discussed the heavily researched validity of the brain-gut connection, as well as the hypothalamic-pituitary-adrenal (HPA) axis response. If gut function is ignored or overlooked in an attempt to heal any of these so-called mental health conditions, the probability of eradicating the illness is very unlikely.

More than one of my patients told me that their medical doctor prescribed Zoloft or Prozac for their digestive problems, when perhaps a simple digestive enzyme may have helped. Enzymes are necessary for every function in the body, including digesting, absorbing, transporting, metabolizing, and eliminating food waste from the diet. The body must have an adequate supply of all enzymes to operate properly and remain healthy. The parasympathetic nervous system, as part of the autonomic nervous system, stimulates the release of digestive enzymes, which means it is automatic. We don't have to think about it. Enzymes are classified into three types: digestive, food, and metabolic.

Digestive enzymes are secreted by the salivary glands, stomach, pancreas, endocrine cells and small intestine, breaking down food to facilitate nutrient absorption from the small and large intestines into the bloodstream.

Food enzymes are present in raw foods, primarily fruits and vegetables, and enter the body with the food. They help digest the food at the time of ingestion and all the way through the digestive tract. This is why it makes sense to eat a salad prior to the main entrée. The enzymes in the raw food assist digestion of cooked foods. Cooked or steamed vegetables and fruits are still healthful for other nutrients; however, cooking and processing foods destroy most of the enzyme content.

Metabolic enzymes benefit all parts of the body and are necessary for the proper functioning of every cell. They act as catalysts to produce energy, remove waste, and detoxify poisons. They are required for new cell growth and to repair and maintain all organs and tissues. Metabolic enzymes also rush to the aid of any inflammatory process in the body.

Let's look at these classes of enzymes and the critical processes each of them provides. From the following, it becomes quite clear that enzyme deficiencies are related to mental and emotional issues as well as fatigue.

Amylase digests carbohydrates and starches as well as dead white blood cells (pus). It is a digestive enzyme that comes from either the salivary glands or the pancreas. Amylase reduces inflammatory reactions, such as those caused by the release of histamine and similar substances. The symptoms of amylase deficiency include psoriasis, eczema, hives, allergic reactions to bee and bug stings, abscesses, atopic dermatitis, all types of herpes, hypoglycemia, depression, moodiness, allergies, premenstrual syndrome, fatigue, hot flashes, cold hands and feet, neck and shoulder aches, and celiac sprue.

Lipase digests fat and fat-soluble vitamins such as Vitamins A, D, E, and K. The tongue, stomach, pancreas, and bile from the gallbladder are responsible for lipase production and action. Deficiencies can encourage high cholesterol, high triglycerides, and diabetes, and make weight loss very difficult. Lipase-deficient people also have decreased cell permeability, meaning nutrients cannot enter and the waste cannot exit. The symptoms of deficiency are aching feet, arthritis, bladder issues, cystitis, acne, gallbladder stress, gallstones, hay fever, enlarged prostate, psoriasis, urinary weakness, constipation, diarrhea, and heart problems.

Cellulase breaks down the fiber in our diet. This food enzyme is essential because our bodies do not produce it. Only raw foods contain cellulase. Of all the enzymes, a deficiency in this one carries with it the most problems. They can be best described as malabsorption syndrome or impaired absorption of nutrients, vitamins, or minerals by the small intestine. Indications for malabsorption may include lower abdominal gas, bloating, and complaints associated with the small intestine and pancreas. Diverticulitis, high cholesterol, irritable bowel syndrome, constipation, hemorrhoids, heart disease, and malnutrition can also manifest.

Sucrase breaks down sucrose, a carbohydrate (sugar). Sucrose-intolerant people cannot split the sucrose disaccharide into two units of glucose required for energy. Glucose is the primary brain food, so this deficiency can cause mental and emotional illness, including depression, moodiness, panic attacks, manic and schizophrenic behavior, and severe mood swings.

Lactase breaks down the lactose sugar in dairy products. Lactose-intolerant people have abdominal cramps, diarrhea, asthma, and other allergic reactions.

Maltase also breaks down sugars. Maltose-intolerant people are generally sensitive to rapid environmental changes and have deficiencies in all other enzymes. Symptoms are Crohn's disease, celiac disease, cramps, diarrhea, and severe allergies.

Protease is one of the primary food enzymes, which digests protein. The many proteases (also called proteolytic enzymes) are derived from animals (and some plants), usually from their pancreas, stomach, or intestine. The word proteolytic means the splitting of proteins by hydrolysis. Proteases cannot digest all foods because they need specific pH to be utilized. Animal enzymes work better in an alkaline solution, which is found in the small intestine. Since the amino acid structure of protein is a major building block of the whole body, the production of protease is critical for all functions and cellular make-up. Protease has the ability to digest unwanted debris in the blood, including certain bacteria and viruses. This enzyme supports immune function and eliminates toxic waste that might develop anywhere in the body. In addition, since protease is required to carry protein-bound calcium in the blood, a protease deficiency lays the foundation for arthritis, osteoporosis, and other calcium-deficiency diseases. The symptoms of protease deficiency are back weakness, constipation, high blood pressure, insomnia, impaired hearing, parasites, gum disorders, cancer, and kidney ailments.

The following are examples of proteolytic enzymes or proteases:

Bromelain is a substance of proteolytic and milk-clotting enzymes derived from pineapple, papayas, mangoes, and kiwis. In concentration these enzymes act as anti-inflammatory agents.

Trypsin is an enzyme formed in the duodenum (lower part of the stomach) and can be taken from the intestine or pancreas of an animal. Trypsin breaks down the amino acids arginine and lysine. This enzyme is used to fortify the pancreas and the acid environment of the large intestine.

Chymotrypsin is a protease variety that aids in breaking down protein. This enzyme is available in supplemental form from bovine or porcine pancreas. Chymotrypsin treats soft tissue injuries and aids in surgical recovery.

Pepsin is a proteolytic enzyme that is usually prepared from pig's stomach. Pepsin's main function is to break down proteins in the stomach. It does not break down carbohydrate or fat.

Pancreatin is a substance taken from the pancreas of an ox or hog. This protease enzyme contains amylase and lipase, and breaks down food best in an alkaline setting (8.0 pH). Accordingly, pancreatin is only effective in the alkaline environment of the small intestine.

Hydrochloric Acid is not usually referred to as an enzyme, but it can break down protein and carbohydrates in the stomach, where it is manufactured. Deficiency of hydrochloric acid will manifest in symptoms like gas, bloating, muscle-wasting or atrophy, depression, anxiety, panic attacks, and fatigue. Hydrochloric acid also has the capacity to kill parasites, H pylori, E coli, and other pathogens.

You can see that what may appear to be so-called simple indigestion can wreak major havoc in the body, gradually deteriorating major organs and systems including the brain and central nervous system. Insufficient enzyme production by the body can be supplemented through high-quality enzyme formulations.

Chart of Enzyme Relationships

Enzyme	Function	Deficiency Symptoms
Amylase	Digests carbohydrates and debris of white blood cells	Skin problems, hypoglycemia, depression, allergies, PMS, fatigue, moodiness, hot flashes, cold hands and feet
Lipase	Digests fat and fat-soluble vitamins	Aching feet, arthritis, high cholesterol, cystitis, anxiety, acne, gallbladder issues, hay fever, constipation, diarrhea, heart and prostate ailments, depression
Cellulase	Breaks down fiber, including raw foods	Malabsorption syndrome (including all GI problems), heart disease, and high cholesterol
Sucrase	Breaks down sucrose carbohydrate	Mental and emotional illnesses such as depression, bipolar disorder, panic attacks, and gluten intolerance
Lactase	Breaks down lactose, the sugar in dairy products	Asthma, allergies, gluten intolerance, irritable bowel, and diarrhea
Maltase	Breaks down sugars	Deficiencies in all other enzymes. Crohn's, celiac, and allergies
Proteolytic (proteases): pancreatin, trypsin, bromelain, chymotrypsin, pepsin	Digests food protein and metabolic waste	Back weakness, high blood pressure, insomnia, hearing impairment, parasites, kidney issues, fungus, constipation, gum disorders, and cancers

Chart of Enzyme Relationships
(Continued)

Enzyme	Function	Deficiency Symptoms
Hydrochloric Acid	Digests protein and carbohydrate	Gas, bloating, distaste for meat, bad breath, body odor, asthma, headaches, reflux, intestinal parasites, and food poisoning

Dietary Changes for Recovery & Locked-In Healing

Forensic Nutrition

Dietary intake is extremely important to rebuilding gut health. Keep in mind that your body is a chemistry lab. What you put into it either supports health or interferes with the body's on-going attempt to heal or remain healthy.

By now, you've seen how the brain-gut connection is vitally important as a biochemical pathway for mental, emotional, and spiritual health. So the subject of nutrition encompasses not only food you ingest, but how that food impacts your health. In fact, every single food should be considered not only as it involves nutrition, but how it contributes to the functional medicine paradigm. I like to think of this as forensic nutrition. For example, the following questions apply equally to a blueberry, a bagel, a carrot, a hamburger, an avocado, olive oil, or a potato chip:

1. Is it acid or alkaline-forming?
2. What is its protein, fat, and carbohydrate content?
3. What is its vitamin and mineral content?
4. Does it contain gluten?
5. Is it organically grown?

6. Is it genetically modified (GMO)?
7. Will it affect yeast and fungus already present in the body?
8. Is it commonly allergy-producing?
9. Is it high in salicylates/phenols (naturally occurring chemicals to which some individuals are sensitive)?
10. What is its oxalate content (a naturally occurring chemical that, if not converted properly by the body, can form crystals in some individuals)?
11. What is its glycemic index; how will it affect blood sugar?
12. Does it contain caffeine?
13. Does it contain saturated or trans-fat?
14. Does it exacerbate current health issues?
15. Does it support long-term health?

Answering these questions can be overwhelming, so finding a qualified health care professional can help. But the bottom line is how you answer questions 14 and 15, above.

Food is, of course, a necessity—it's not only the fuel on which your body runs, it's also required to replenish, recover, and restore. Eating whole, clean, live foods will dictate the difference in how you feel, how you think, how you act, and how you look. Eating a continual diet of junk food, fast food, and fake food is not only unhealthy physically, but can depress and dull the mind as well.

Since your body requires an array of different vitamins, minerals, amino acids, fats, proteins, carbohydrates, and other nutrients, it needs a variety of different foods to meet those requirements. A common reason many people overeat is to try to meet that need. A life event might create a deficit, which in turn creates a physiological need for food high in a particular nutrient, such a Vitamin C. A physiological need or true hunger for fat or salt is not satisfied by eating cucumbers and carrots. Your body might crave fat because of a fatty acid imbalance or if there is disruption in the liver and gallbladder, which help to digest and absorb fat. True hunger can also stem from incomplete digestion or absorption of a critical

A physiological need or true hunger for fat or salt is not satisfied by eating cucumbers and carrots.

nutrient, or not getting it in your diet, or as a supplement.

Nutrient deficiencies also result from a monotonous diet and increase cravings. Sugar, for instance, is a very addictive substance that interferes with serotonin and other neurotransmitter receptors in the brain. Sugar is addictive for a variety of reasons that were discussed in Part Four, "Donuts and Road Rage." I'm not just picking on donuts, I am calling out all sugar and fake-sugar chemicals as substances more prevalent than any other ingredient in the modern American diet that negatively impact the body, especially the brain and its cognitive processes. The food you eat creates mixtures of chemical responses that affect our bodies in either healthful or harmful ways.

Food and Psychology

In our society today, food and drink serve many purposes. You may grab a donut and a cup of coffee first thing in the morning to give you a quick energy boost, or a soft drink and a candy bar mid-afternoon to help you stay awake, alert, and focused on finishing the project that's due at five o'clock. You might eat a bowl of cereal before you go to bed to help you get to sleep.

Many people eat to numb painful memories or to avoid experiencing painful or unpleasant emotions such as fear, depression, anger, boredom, rejection, or loneliness. Although food is meant to nourish our physical bodies, as emotive human beings, we are apt to use food for nurturing as well. Even healthy foods are commonly eaten in excess, as mentioned earlier, to help fill a nutrient void. Proverbs 25:16 reads: "Have you found honey? Eat only what you need, lest you have it in excess and vomit it."

The food you eat creates mixtures of chemical responses that affect our bodies in either healthful or harmful ways.

Food addictions and abuses such as binge eating, anorexia, and bulimia very commonly have psychological as well as physiological and spiritual associations. Any food (or body) abuses that prompt an individual to eat in the absence of true physical hunger can signify biochemical and nutritional deficits. So-called comfort-food eating, binge eating, and other forms of food addictions are in most cases related to brain chemical neurotransmitter imbalances of s such as serotonin, dopamine, epinephrine, and norepinephrine. Even certain smells that retrieve specific memories can cause chemical imbalances, which in turn influence particular food choices or turn off the appetite entirely. A good example of this occurs in pregnancy when chemical and hormonal imbalances cause cravings for specific foods or nausea in response to particular aromas.

About fifteen years ago I was roasting two bulbs of garlic in my oven (something I had never done before) to make a healthy version of a recipe I found in a magazine. The aroma was heavenly! About thirty minutes through the roasting process, and seemingly out of nowhere, I developed a violent stomach virus that lasted about twenty-four hours. Needless to say, I never finished that recipe. That experience created a strong aversion to roasted garlic. These days, when a recipe calls for roasted garlic, I substitute fresh pressed garlic or leave it out altogether. My logical brain is protecting my body from going through that same awful experience now associated with that aroma. Of course, I can retrain my brain. But if I can use garlic that I don't have to roast and still get the same health benefits, why create another stressor? Interestingly, about three years after the garlic fiasco, I discovered (through IgG food allergy testing) that I have a moderately delayed allergy to garlic.

The brain-gut connection, the HPA stress response of the adrenal glands, and the complex interactions between the hormonal, neurotransmitter, and central nervous messaging systems are all involved in food choices, aversions, addictions or other food-related behaviors. The amazing chemistry lab that God created is surely

Your thoughts and word choices about your behaviors also affect how your body responds.

more complicated, than even the most brilliant scientists can comprehend.

Your thoughts and word choices about yourself also affect your body responses. Constantly using language like, "I cheated", "I screwed up today", or "I'll just quit" are negative, damaging, and defeating words that are not profitable for healing. The important thing is to recognize how you use food and to make intelligent choices about your behavior toward food. Being a fanatic is not necessary, especially if you feel you are in good health. Just make wise choices most of the time. You can choose not to use food to nurture, or you can make a conscious choice to occasionally use food to nurture and acknowledge that you are okay with it. Regard your body as a temple where the Holy Spirit of God resides (1 Corinthians 3: 16). Keep your temple clean and pure physically, mentally, and spiritually.

Becoming aware of your emotional connections to eating is important. But realize, also, that satan and his minions want nothing more than to mess with your mind and convince you that you will never be good enough, you will never overcome your addictions, or any number of other crushing and conquering words to continue to beat you down. For the healing process to continue, you must realize that God is your victorious warrior and He has ultimate power. You possess that power, too, if His Spirit lives in you by salvation through His Son, Jesus Christ. I love what Beth Moore said about self-control in *Living Beyond Yourself*:

> "The key to self-control is the refusal to allow our enemies (the flesh, the world or Satan) to rule or hold us captive in any way. Self-control is our wall of protection. Our lack of self-control makes us vulnerable to attack from the enemy. Christ has given us the victory over our flesh, our world, and our accuser … They cannot presume authority over us."

In order for the healing process to continue, you must realize that God is your victorious warrior and that He has ultimate power.

Finally, making dietary lifestyle changes include changing not only what and why you eat, but how you eat as well. For example, use all five senses to enjoy your food, not just the sense of taste. The senses of smell, sight, hearing, and touch, also enhance the enjoyment of eating. As you experience daily improvement in feelings of anxiety, depression, and fatigue, you will also begin to notice improvement in other areas, such as allergies, asthma, skin conditions, and digestive issues. Symptoms can be totally eliminated while healing is accomplished at the cellular level using a complete nutritional approach. The digestive tract promotes far more than good digestion—total health hangs in the balance.

Bad-Mood Foods

To support the detoxification and healing process to overcome depression, anxiety, and fatigue, avoid the following foods and items that pretend to be food. They deplete valuable vitamins, minerals, good bacteria, and other nutrients and further interfere with your body's ability to heal itself.

- Any food or drink to which you are addicted
- Coffee, black tea, and alcohol
- Fruit juices
- All fruits (except grapefruit, lemons, limes, Granny Smith apples, and all berries). Do not eat dried fruits.
- White flour and wheat, rye and barley flours
- Sugar and all foods containing sugar
- All dairy products (except organic butter or ghee-clarified butter)

- Corn and corn products
- Peanuts and peanut butter
- All vinegars (except unpasteurized apple cider vinegar)
- Hydrogenated or partially hydrogenated fats, corn or soybean oil and charbroiled meats
- Chemical sugar substitutes like high-fructose corn syrup, sucralose also known as Splenda, aspartame also known as Equal, NutraSweet, agave syrup, honey, molasses, maple, rice, and other syrups
- Soy and soy-containing foods (excluding fermented soy, such as miso or tempeh, or organic and non-GMO edamame beans)
- Commercially prepared fried foods
- Farmed fish or Atlantic or Pacific caught
- Packaged foods containing MSG (monosodium glutamate), preservatives, additives, colorings, aluminum, or mercury

After the detoxification program and when you feel more stable and healthy, but no sooner than six weeks add back in other fruits, modest amounts of peanut butter and non-GMO corn products, and other vinegars such as balsamic. Locally grown honey, non-sulphured molasses, Grade B (now referred to as "Grade A, dark amber, robust taste") maple syrup, and rice syrup may be used in modest amounts, as well as some dried fruit.

Good-Mood Foods

Sources of nutrients to support gastrointestinal health and recovery are found in:

Protein—such as fish and their oils. Wild-caught Alaskan and Norwegian are preferable because of their negligible mercury content. My long-time preference for purchasing fish is from www.VitalChoice.com. Grass-fed organic meats, poultry, and eggs. Organic plain and Greek yogurt (for some cow-sourced yogurt should be temporarily eliminated). Goat and sheep milk yogurt can be tolerated by most. Goat and sheep cheeses. Pea or rice protein powders.

Fats—such as organic, extra-virgin oils: coconut oil, olive oil, macadamia nut oil, walnut oil, and grapeseed oil. Organic butter or ghee (clarified butter). Seeds such as sesame, pumpkin, chia, and flax. Nuts: pecan, walnut, almond, Brazil, macadamia, cashew, and their butters.

Carbohydrates—Low-carbohydrate vegetables such as the green, leafy variety and fruits (preferably organic and non-GMO) are mineral-dense and tend to be alkalinizing for the body. Eating too many low carbohydrate vegetables is pretty difficult. Higher carbohydrate and root vegetables including potatoes, carrots, artichokes, ginger, radishes, beets, and yams are nutrient dense, too. Fresh is always best, but frozen is fine. Avoid canned vegetables and fruits. Legumes such as lentils, beans, and peas. Quinoa, brown or basmati rice, gluten-free oatmeal, or other gluten-free, minimally processed foods, like brown rice flour tortillas.

Other good-mood foods—such as coconut milk, rice milk or almond milk. Herbal teas can be emotionally soothing. And don't forget about cultured and fermented vegetables, quinoa milk, coconut water, or coconut milk.

Genetically Modified Foods (GMO)

Do you have any idea if the strawberries you ate for breakfast this morning were spliced with fish genes? Or were the green beans you planned for dinner this evening genetically altered using pig parts? Many chemical companies, such as Monsanto, have been experimenting with genetic modification—yes, manipulating the genetic structure of common, ordinary food—for more than twenty-five years. The first genetically modified food, the Flavr SavrTM tomato, hit store shelves in 1994. Incidentally, twenty percent of the research mice force-fed these tomatoes died within two weeks.

So, what's the purpose of genetic modification? These crops, which now include corn, canola, wheat, alfalfa, cotton, and sorghum, begin with a seed that is genetically split or modified and referred to as "Roundup Ready" to make the crop resistant to the herbicide Roundup (manufactured by Monsanto), which is used to kill weeds in the farmers' fields. The active ingredient in Roundup is glyphosate, one of the most toxic chemicals known to mankind.

Today, Monsanto and other chemical companies are working on pest-resistant bananas, high-yield black-eyed peas, and millet immune to parasitic infection. These might sound like great goals, but we are being used as human experiments while these chemical companies profit from patented technology and increased seed and chemical sales. Gene splicing can cause serious problems, among them new food allergies. Imagine eating seemingly healthy green beans when your throat starts to swell because you're allergic to pork! Other serious problems:

- Pollution from these airborne chemicals and genetic microorganisms
- Major antibiotic resistance
- New diseases and illnesses yet to be named

Did you think Mad Cow Disease was a freak of nature? The unintended consequences are real and quite frightening. Unfortunately, the FDA does not yet require these foods to be labeled as genetically modified. The environmental and health risks are enormous.

My GMO Tomato Story

About ten years ago, I went to the grocery to purchase produce for a salad to take to a party to which I was invited. I selected all organic produce, except the tomatoes (because the store was out of them). I assembled all the ingredients into a luscious salad, using only one of the three beautiful, bright red, commercially grown "tomatoes-on-the-vine" I had purchased. I left the remaining two on the counter for future use.

After two weeks, the tomatoes on the counter remained as beautiful as they were when I purchased them. As more weeks passed, they still "looked vibrant and fresh" and I was becoming fearful of what we had eaten. Finally, after two months, a soft spot appeared on those "things." Folks, those were not tomatoes! I don't know what they were, but I will never buy another non-organic, non-GMO tomato again, and neither should you. If research mice died within two weeks after being force-fed GMO food, then certainly our sustained long-term health depends on staying away from these franken-foods.

The best way to avoid genetically modified foods is to buy organic. To meet USDA organic standards, a genetically modified seed or crop may not be used. Organic produce uses a 5-digit PLU sticker number prefaced by a number 9.

Stay away from processed foods, as well, especially those using the GMO crops mentioned above. Look for the label "Non-GMO" and "Organic" on minimally processed or packaged foods.

If research mice died within two weeks of being force-fed GMO food, then certainly our sustained long-term health depends on staying away from these franken-foods.

Below is a list of the top twelve produce that should always be purchased organic due to the amount of pesticides used during growing. The lowest number indicates the highest amount of pesticide:

1. Strawberries
2. Apples
3. Nectarines
4. Peaches
5. Celery
6. Grapes
7. Cherries
8. Spinach
9. Tomatoes
10. Sweet Bell Peppers
11. Cherry Tomatoes
12. Cucumbers

The following foods have the lowest pesticide load, and therefore can be purchased commercially grown. However, if they're not organic then they are potentially GMO. You may find more information on the Environmental Working Group website, www.ewg.org.

1. Avocados
2. Sweet corn
3. Pineapples
4. Cabbage
5. Sweet peas
6. Onions
7. Asparagus
8. Mangoes
9. Papayas
10. Kiwi
11. Eggplant
12. Honeydew
13. Grapefruit
14. Cantaloupe
15. Cauliflower

Gluten and Gluten-Free Foods

Gluten should definitely be avoided to return the body to optimal health. Gluten is the protein or polypeptide found predominately in wheat, rye, and barley grains. These grains are found in baked goods and most packaged and processed foods, which constitute a large percentage of the daily American diet. Bulgur, couscous, farina, kamut, spelt, and semolina are other grains that contain gluten. Gluten can also be hidden in canned soups, seasoning packets, salad dressings, marinades, soy sauce, malt flavorings, and others packaged foods. Even rice syrup is sometimes made with barley malt. In some fast food restaurants, gluten is used in the seasoned salt on French fries to get the salt to stick.

Quinoa, buckwheat, teff, amaranth, millet, and tapioca are good examples of naturally gluten-free grains that can be included in the diet, as long as they are not combined with other gluten-containing grains. Reading labels on so-called gluten-free packaged foods is also important. On the ingredient label, the manufacturer will disclose whether sugar, malt, yeast, or other unhealthy items have been added. These should also be avoided.

Whey, Casein, and Lactose

Whey and casein are proteins found in all dairy products. Lactose is the milk sugar. Generally speaking, an individual who is "allergic" to lactose will be sensitive to whey and casein, as well. Of all the food allergy tests I conducted over the last twenty years, every single individual exhibited an intolerance to whey, and most to casein, as well. Consider for a minute that many cows are grain-fed instead of grass-fed, so they produce milk containing gliadin/gluten. As the preceding chapters have discussed, food allergies or intolerances to gluten aggravate the immune system, creating an inflammatory cascade culminating in depression and anxiety.

Sugar

The most recent research in 2015 shows that the average person consumes 32 teaspoons of sugar per day ...

Enough can never be said about the challenges to maintaining physical and mental health while yet consuming sugar. The most recent research in 2015 shows that the average person consumes 32 teaspoons of sugar per day according to a study by Euromonitor (a London-based market research firm). This is equivalent to 128 grams per day (1 teaspoon = 4 grams). Sugar and sugar-containing foods increase the metabolic load on the body and create an acidic condition, which not only creates but also drives inflammation.

To help alleviate sugar cravings, which are typical in a body out of homeostasis, the amino acid l-glutamine is very helpful. L-glutamine also supports healing of the gut lining and prevents breakdown of lean muscle mass. See Part Six, Detoxification to Prevent Foundational Stages of Disease for more information on eliminating fungus and other pathogens that contribute to sugar cravings.

Chemical Sweeteners

Chemical sugar substitutes like Splenda (trademark name for sucralose), Equal (trademark name for aspartame), NutraSweet (another trademark name for aspartame and neotame) have been implicated in brain lesions, liver damage, seizures, panic attacks, headaches, blindness, birth defects, and many other illnesses. As if those aren't scary enough, research has also shown that NutraSweet kills good bacteria in the gut.

Soy

Fermented soy products should only be used if they are non-GMO and organic. Examples are tempeh, miso, and some tofu and edamame. Common foodstuffs today contain too much processed soy, which can interfere with thyroid and other hormones as well as enzyme function. The soy manufacturing process utilizes large aluminum vats from which the metal leaches into the soy and further burdens the body with heavy metals.

Cultured and Fermented Foods

Jonathan Lamb, a humanities professor at Vanderbilt University, conducted extensive research over the years on the disease of scurvy, a severe depletion of Vitamin C. His research includes how diseases of malnutrition prevalent in the 18th Century, including scurvy and rickets (severe vitamin D deficiency) could have been prevented. He authored the book, *Scurvy: The Disease of Discovery,* in which he describes how Captain James Cook carried aboard one of his sailing vessels almost 8,000 pounds of sauerkraut—cabbage finely chopped and fermented in its own natural juice—which prevented these diseases in his sailors.

Cultured and fermented foods help to re-establish the healthy terrain and environment of the gastrointestinal tract. In addition to probiotic growth, the cultured and fermented foods will nurture many vitamins, minerals, lactoferrin, and peptides providing antimicrobial and antioxidant properties.

Cultured foods can be made at home easily by shredding or chopping cabbage or other vegetables and packing them tightly in an air-tight glass or stainless steel container. They will slowly ferment over five or six days at room temperature, then can be stored in the refrigerator as long as twelve months. Enjoy a forkful daily with one of your meals. Starter cultures are not necessary but can be used to ensure a more hearty strain of healthy bacteria (probiotic).

Research has shown fermented foods to be valuable for anxiety and depression, as well as their influence on brain health, directly or indirectly through the gut. One scientific author commented that "… the borderline between food and medicine is becoming very thin."

Some examples of fermented or cultured foods include sauerkraut, which is made by fermenting cabbage. Kimchi is a Korean staple made by fermenting cabbage with other vegetables. Kombucha is a fermented sweet tea with bacteria cultures. Kefir, fermented cow's milk similar to yogurt, is very beneficial for supporting gastrointestinal health and generally better tolerated than yogurt.

Other foods that can be fermented are coconut water, quinoa, fish, or other meat. Individuals with gut issues such as SIBO (small intestinal bacterial overgrowth) may not tolerate these foods well, initially. You can find more information about cultured and fermented foods and purchase starters at http://www.bodyecology.com.

Rebuilding With Micronutrient Supplementation

Supplements were never intended to be a magic pill. Many times I've told my clients, "If they were, I'd give you one and take two myself!" I only recommend a supplement (typically herbal, homeopathic, or magnesium) in severe cases to alleviate the symptom while digging into the root cause. Taking a supplement for a symptom only differs from taking a drug in that supplements typically produce no negative side effects. The purpose of supplements is just what the name implies—to supplement food intake with additional nutrition for the body to remain stable or improve health. Our bodies are very dynamic. As such, the same nutrient is not intended for long-term intake, except for a high-quality vitamin and mineral complex, or in cases of genetic polymorphism like MTHF-R where the human body cannot manufacture a particular nutrient, or the diet remains insufficient.

Why Take Supplements?

Over the years, I have been asked and re-asked these two questions: Is it true that dietary supplements are not regulated, and why take them in the first place?

The FDA and FTC do have significant regulatory authority over dietary supplements. Unlike drugs, however, no pre-approval is required for vitamins and supplements because they are commonly found in food and have a much safer profile than drugs. The FDA requires compliance with meat and poultry companies, as well.

The FTC (Federal Trade Commission), enforces the FDA and asserts its authority frequently to ensure truthful and prevent misleading labeling. The vast majority of infractions are against direct-to-consumer companies. To my knowledge, the FTC has not conducted a single action on products sold exclusively through qualified health care practitioners' offices.

Products offered by a healthcare practitioner should be the most researched and highest quality products available. A good healthcare provider should stay current on the latest research. They should actually visit the manufacturing facilities where products carrying the FDA required cGMP (current Good Manufacturing Practice) seal are produced. Purchasing supplements from a qualified healthcare provider that you trust and who satisfies these criteria is critically preferable to purchasing on-line or in a big-box store.

Every once in a while as my clients report dramatic health improvement to their physicians through nutritional therapies, supplements, and dietary protocols, the physician will respond one of two ways—attribute the improvement to spontaneous remission or recommend my client keep doing what they're doing—when the physician has not the slightest interest in actually knowing what the client did. Some clients also report that their primary care physicians see no reason to take supplements. Of course, I strongly disagree on many grounds, but here are two key reasons:

1. Industrialized nations lead incredibly stressful lives that deplete nutrients critical for the body to function properly, like sleeping well, having good, stable energy and brain function, detoxing properly, and keeping hormones and gut balanced, among others.

2. Many people eat the same things over and over, day in and day out. A wide variety of foods is required to replete all the necessary nutrients. But even if we get a variety, foods today are lacking in minerals, genetically modified, chemically preserved, colored, or sweetened, and overloaded with pesticides.

Taking dietary supplements is now more important than ever. Many traditional dietitians and others of the medical mindset believe we can get enough vitamins and minerals from our foods and beverages. This mentality is contradicted by the research. In addition to the highly processed, standard American diet, foods are stored for long periods of time—you may as well eat cardboard—and many people have zero desire to eat whole, fresh, live, natural foods. Seasonal variation and even personal selection of foods contribute to nutrient inadequacies, not to mention the harmful effects of some extreme fad diets.

Taking dietary supplements is now more important than ever.

The RDA (recommended daily/dietary allowance), originally established in the 1940s by the United States National Academy of Sciences, was designed with the intent of eliminating severe nutrient deficiency diseases such as beriberi (vitamin B1 deficiency), pellagra (vitamin B3 deficiency), and scurvy (vitamin C deficiency). However, RDA standards have never considered the impact of our highly polluted environment, chlorinated and fluoridated drinking water, herbicides, pesticides, phthalates, and the lifestyles we lead, which include stress, smoking, alcohol, antacids, birth control pills, aspirin, and laxatives.

Prescription and over-the-counter drug use are more prevalent than ever before. Drugs both interfere with nutrient absorption and elevate normal nutrient requirements. As you have seen from the discussions on adrenal burnout and fatigue, stress also depletes nutrients by creating huge demands on certain vitamins and minerals in amounts that are impossible to replace from food alone. These are risky combinations and do not support the allopathic mindset for balanced health from food alone.

Furthermore, since the body cannot manufacture some nutrients, they must be supplied by either your diet or from supplements. Even some of the B vitamins, which are manufactured in the intestine, might be unavailable due to inadequate friendly probiotic bacteria, lack of intrinsic factor, a substance produced in the stomach which helps to absorb B12, or lymph congestion anywhere in the body. The lack of proper vitamins, minerals, and other nutrients over a prolonged period results in serious and distressing health problems exacerbated when the body attempts to compensate in further destructive ways. For example, a serious lack of choline, an essential nutrient found in beans and eggs, will force the body to compensate by eating its own brain tissue and nervous system.

Drugs both interfere with nutrient absorption and elevate normal requirements of nutrients.

Thousands upon thousands of studies, including double-blind, placebo-controlled research, show stabilizing or recovery benefits of many herbal and rainforest nutrients such as St. John's Wort, rhodiola, ginseng, Pau D'Arco, berberine, saffron, golden seal, garlic, cat's claw, feverfew, Echinacea, and countless others. These nutrients alone or in combinations, have many far reaching uses and side benefits without the actual harmful side effects of pharmaceutical preparations.

Whether your diagnosis is CFIDS (chronic fatigue immune dysfunction syndrome), fibromyalgia, rheumatoid arthritis, depression, anxiety, or cancer, the plethora of research studies both current and having endured over the years on omega-3 fatty acids, S-Adenosyl-L-Methionine (SAMe), probiotics, glutamine, N-acetyl cysteine, minerals, B vitamins, and many others, offers an inordinate variety of opportunities to support recovery in natural ways.

Vitamins

Did you know that vitamins and minerals do not contribute directly toward energy? Rather, they are micronutrient co-factors essential for the release of energy from macronutrients called protein, fat, and carbohydrate that you consume. In other words, vitamins and minerals work together synergistically with food to provide ideal energy utilization by the body. Low levels of specific micronutrients will prevent absorption of other micro and macronutrients.

The B vitamins, in particular, are very important to the central nervous system to combat fatigue, depression, and anxiety. B vitamins are sometimes referred to as the psychiatric vitamins because of their importance as precursor nutrients in brain function and production of neurotransmitters. See the chart on Amino Acids and Brain Function in Part Six. Nutrients in the body are like dominoes standing on end in a neat row several feet in length. Gently tapping the first one causes the entire row to cascade perfectly. Now remove one here and there. The "cascade" will never be accomplished properly because of the missing dominoes. Likewise, vitamins and minerals depend on one another to carry out the many metabolic and chemical cascades that must occur in the body to provide optimal health.

Consider tryptophan, which makes 5HTP, which then makes serotonin. Also, tyrosine makes L-Dopa, which then makes dopamine. Tryptophan and tyrosine are amino acids mainly supplied from protein-containing food. Each of these major conversions requires precursor nutrients and enzymes for completion. In these cases of neurotransmitter transfer, iron, magnesium, B6, SAMe, copper, Vitamin C, and other nutrients are required.

The purpose of vitamins is to form complex chemical compounds in the body, which engage in enzymatic activity necessary to convert food to energy, to build tissue, and to prevent damage from free radical (toxic) activity in the body. The mere act of moving an arm or leg or even deep concentration creates free radical activity in the body, which pales in comparison to the enormous free radical activity created by chemicals, parasites, viruses, bacteria, heavy metals, and the polluted environment. Getting the necessary vitamins as noted on the following chart is extremely important to all aspects of physical, emotional, and mental health.

Water Soluble Vitamins

Essential Nutrients	Signs of Deficiency	Prevents Absorption	Supports Absorption	Food Sources
B1—Thiamine	Depression, constipation, weakness, fatigue	Alcohol, tobacco, caffeine, fever, stress, surgery, raw clams	Vitamins C, B-complex, folic acid, E, and manganese	Dairy products, organ meats, brewer's yeast
B2—Riboflavin	Dermatitis, sore tongue, poor digestion, inflammation of mouth, eye disorders	Alcohol, tobacco, caffeine, excessive sugar	Vitamins C, B-complex, and phosphorus	Dairy products, organ meats, brewer's yeast, fish eggs, beans
B3—Niacin	Loss of appetite, insomnia, depression, muscle aches, GI ailments	Alcohol, caffeine, excessive sugar, corn	Vitamins C, B-complex, and phosphorus	Wheat germ, fish, poultry, desiccated liver
B5—Pantothenic Acid	Hypoglycemia, hair loss, fatigue, vomiting, diarrhea, insulin sensitivity	Caffeine, alcohol	Vitamins C, B-complex, folic acid, biotin, and sulfur	Organ meats, brewer's yeast
B6—Pyridoxine	Nervousness, hair loss, insulin sensitivity, acne, irritability, muscle weakness, depression	Alcohol, tobacco, caffeine, birth control pills, radiation	Vitamin B-complex, and magnesium, sodium, and essential fatty acid	Meats, fish, whole grains, broccoli, legumes, spinach

Water Soluble Vitamins

(Continued)

Essential Nutrients	Signs of Deficiency	Prevents Absorption	Supports Absorption	Food Sources
B12—Cobalamin	General weakness and fatigue, poor appetite, pernicious anemia, nervousness	Alcohol, tobacco, caffeine, laxatives, lack of hydrochloric acid	Vitamins B-complex, folic acid, and choline, inositol, and potassium	Eggs, meat, fish, poultry, dairy, brewer's yeast
Folic Acid	B-12 deficiency, cardiovascular diseases, anemia, gray hair	Alcohol, tobacco, caffeine, stress	Vitamins C, B-complex, biotin	Wheat germ, beans, peas, green leafy vegetables
Biotin	Extreme exhaustion, depression, gray skin color, inability to metabolize fat, diabetes	Alcohol, caffeine, raw egg white	Vitamins C, B-complex, folic acid, and sulfur	Lamb, liver, egg yolks, nuts
Inositol	High cholesterol, constipation, skin afflictions, eye disorders, depression	Alcohol, caffeine, antibiotics, corn, excessive sugar	Vitamins C, B-complex, choline, and essential fatty acids	Whole grains, liver, lecithin
Choline	Fatty liver, ulcers, high blood pressure	Alcohol, caffeine, excessive sugar	Vitamins A, B-complex, biotin, folic acid, and essential fatty acid	Egg yolks, lecithin

Fat Soluble Vitamins

Essential Nutrients	Signs of Deficiency	Prevents Absorption	Supports Absorption	Food Sources
Vitamin A	Teeth and gum problems, allergies, eye disorders, dry skin, loss of smell	Alcohol, caffeine, excessive iron, vitamin D deficiency	Vitamins C, D, E, B-complex, choline and calcium, zinc	Carrots, liver, eggs, cod liver oil, cream, fruit
Vitamin D	Rickets, muscle weakness, malabsorption of calcium, diarrhea, insomnia, soft teeth and bones	Mineral oil	Vitamins A, C, choline, and phosphorus, calcium, and essential fatty acids	Sunlight, cod liver oil, egg yolk, fish
Vitamin E	Weak red blood cells, dry skin and hair, heart disease, male and female reproductive difficulties	Mineral oil, birth control pills, chlorine	Vitamins A, C, B-complex, inositol, and selenium, manganese, and essential fatty acids,	Cold-pressed oils, sweet potatoes, almonds, walnuts, spinach
Vitamin K	Blood's inability to clot, malabsorption, nose bleeds, miscarriages	Mineral oil, X-rays, aspirin, rancid fat	Probiotics and healthy gut	Leafy green vegetables, tomatoes, liver, carrots

Minerals

Vitamins cannot function without minerals, and mineral imbalances in the body are a key factor for a poor microbiome as well as energy depletion. Vitamins are like the gas in your car, and minerals are like the spark plugs that ignite the fuel.

Vitamins are like the gas in your car, and minerals are like the spark plugs which ignite the fuel.

My friend, Patty, and I chuckled as she told me this story. Her husband had purchased a bottle of magnesium gel to apply topically for aching muscles and to increase his magnesium stores. He took the bottle into the bathroom, and for reasons unknown to her, he did not turn on a light, even though the room was mostly dark. He shook the bottle before application, opened the lid, and had a beautiful fireworks display! The pressure from shaking had caused the mineral gel to explode upon release creating incredible sparks of energy. I believe that God allows us these experiences just to remind us of how miraculously He created our bodies.

If foundational minerals are missing from the body, toxic metals such as cadmium, aluminum, mercury, lead, and arsenic can replace them in enzyme binding sites throughout the body. Toxic metals contribute to a wide range of health conditions from anxiety, depression, and fatigue to arthritis and Alzheimer's.

Life is in the blood. Minerals such as calcium, magnesium, sodium, potassium, and other supporting nutrients combine to brew the proper chemical mixture for a healthy, hot wire transfer of messages throughout the brain and central nervous system, including hormones, neurotransmitters, and cardiovascular electricity.

> *For the life of the flesh is in the blood, and I have given it to you on the altar to make atonement for your souls; for it is the blood by reason of the life that makes atonement.*
>
> Leviticus 17:11

Minerals help bodily fluids remain pH stable. If the blood becomes too acidic then the buffer minerals calcium, magnesium, and other alkaline minerals will be pulled out of the bones and teeth naturally to reduce acidity in the blood. You can survive toothless with osteoporosis, but you cannot survive if the blood is too acidic for too long—or too alkaline, for that matter. Stress, weakened or burned-out adrenal glands, a high sugar and carbohydrate diet, fried foods, and carbonated beverages all contribute to an overly-acidic body.

Minerals and Emotions

Minerals are uniquely involved in your body's ability to feel emotion. Every mineral has a reflective effect on mental and emotional health and, is thereby, expressly linked to anxiety, depression, and fatigue.

Calcium—mental and emotional protection
Magnesium—physical and emotional relaxation
Chromium—mental and emotional flexibility
Sodium—emergency energy
Potassium—adaptive energy
Zinc—masculine hormone balance
Copper—feminine hormone balance

Biochemical patterns reflected through hair mineral analysis such as low sodium to potassium ratios, elevated calcium, and depleted magnesium can provide a picture of emotional and mental balance as well as physiological health. For instance, extremely low sodium to potassium ratios reflect adrenal burnout. Under times of great stress, prior to adrenal burnout, just the opposite happens. The adrenal hormone, aldosterone, compromises potassium causing sodium levels to rise, which, in turn causes inflammation since aldosterone is a pro-inflammatory hormone. Elevated hair copper combined with low magnesium usually confirms anxiety due to hormonal imbalances.

Mineral Status of our Produce

Vegetables and fruits contain nowhere near the number of nutrients they once contained even as recently as fifty years ago. Good commercial farming practices such as crop rotation are no longer common. The idea of rotating crops was meant to increase soil fertility and discourage pests and disease. The soil is depleted of many minerals after years of growing seasons without replenishing the earth through crop rotation. Awareness of the benefits of allowing the land to lay fallow dates back to at least Biblical times, where the land rested for one year every seven years.

> *You shall sow your land for six years and gather in its yield, but on the seventh year you shall let it rest and lie fallow, so that the needy of your people may eat; and whatever they leave the beast of the field may eat. You are to do the same with your vineyard and your olive grove.*
>
> Exodus 23:10-11

The mineral content of our crops was the subject of a recent study at Rutgers University. The study compared organically grown vegetables with those commercially grown and revealed some astonishing facts regarding minerals.

Results for two minerals in particular—magnesium and iron—revealed that to equal the magnesium content in one organic tomato it takes twenty-four commercially grown tomatoes, and for one head of organic lettuce, it takes four commercial heads. The iron content of one leaf of organic spinach is equivalent to eighty leaves of commercially grown spinach. And finally, to equal the iron content in one organic tomato, it takes two-thousand commercially grown tomatoes! This research proves the glaring lack of nutrients in our standard food supply today and illustrates the critical need for supplementation, especially minerals, if you are not eating organic produce.

Chart of Minerals

Essential Nutrients	Signs of Deficiency	Prevents Absorption	Supports Absorption	Food Sources
Calcium	Back and leg pain, tooth decay, heart palpitations	Lack of hydrochloric acid, stress, lack of exercise, lack of magnesium and Vitamin D	Vitamins A, C, D, and essential fatty acids, iron	Beans, legumes, leafy greens, almonds, sunflower seeds
Chromium	Insulin stabilization	Excess dietary sugar	Zinc, essential fatty acids	Brewer's yeast, whole grains, oysters, shrimp, beef liver
Iodine	Obesity, irritability, cold hands and feet	None	None	Kelp and other sea vegetables
Iron	Weakness, constipation, brittle nails	Excess phosphorus, caffeine	Vitamins C, B12, folic acid, and phosphorus, copper, calcium,	Kelp, meats, eggs, green vegetables
Magnesium	Anxiety, twitches, tremors, confusion, constipation	None	Vitamins C, D, B-6, and calcium, protein	Green leafy vegetables, molasses, brown rice, almonds, cashews
Manganese	Dizziness, hearing loss	Excessive intake of phosphorus and calcium	Excessive phosphorus and calcium intake	Greens, rhubarb, oatmeal, carrots, eggs, lamb, cantaloupe

Chart of Minerals

(Continued)

Essential Nutrients	Signs of Deficiency	Prevents Absorption	Supports Absorption	Food Sources
Phosphorus	Weight/ appetite loss, fatigue, nervousness, overweight	Excessive intake of aluminum, sugar, and iron	Vitamins A, D and protein, manganese, iron, calcium	Meats, whole grains, green leafy vegetables
Potassium	Cardiovascular diseases, acne, thirst, constipation, dry skin, nervousness, thyroid weakness	Alcohol, caffeine, diuretics, excess sugar, stress, laxatives, cortisone	Vitamin B-6 and sodium	Bananas, oranges, avocado, tomatoes, squash, sunflower seeds
Zinc	Loss of taste, poor appetite, fatigue, delayed growth or sexual maturity, anorexia, eating disorders	Alcohol, high calcium intake and lack of phosphorus	Vitamin A, and copper, calcium, phosphorus	Pumpkin seeds, oysters, lamb, shrimp, parsley
Selenium	Premature aging	None	Vitamin E	Smoked herring, liver, eggs, bran, Brazil nuts

Essential Amino Acids

Amino acids are critical for enzyme function, and enzymes, as we've already seen, are critical for every activity in the human body. Currently, scientists understand the function and importance of only about twenty-one amino acids. Nine of the twenty-one are essential, meaning the body cannot make them—we must ingest them from an outside source. The nine essential amino acids are histidine, lysine, leucine, isoleucine, methionine, phenylalanine, threonine, tryptophan, and valine.

These and other amino acids in the following chart are very important for neurotransmitter function in the brain. Amino acids cause these energetically charged messages (neurotransmitters) to travel from one nerve cell to another, as well as bi-directionally communicate along the gut-brain axis. These brain chemicals are supported by the microbiome of a healthy gut and are critical to the optimal function of the central nervous system, as well as the hormonal system. The fat-soluble vitamin D is also very important to protect these chemical messengers.

The only source of these nine essential amino acids is food containing protein and encapsulated or powdered amino acids. Many vegetarians, but especially vegans, do not consume enough building block amino acids from protein in their diet. As a result they frequently feel tired, wired, depressed, and angry.

Food sources for the precursors listed in the chart that support brain chemicals include:

Zinc—pumpkin seeds, legumes, parsley, spinach, beef, and oysters
B vitamins—seeds, nuts, beans, whole grains, beef
Calcium—almonds, leafy greens, oatmeal, dried figs, beans
Magnesium–leafy greens, seeds, beans, cacao
Essential fatty acids—Fish, fish oil, coconut oil, flax oil, borage oil
Vitamin C—fruits, peppers, watercress, spinach, broccoli

Amino acids are also critical building blocks to repair muscle mass and to support the heart muscle. Amino acids boost brain function and alertness as well as prevent degenerative brain diseases like Alzheimer's and Parkinson's. Because amino acids support neurotransmitter production, they should always be included in a natural health program to relieve fatigue and reverse depression and anxiety.

Amino Acids and Brain Function

Amino Acids	Necessary Precursor	Brain Chemical or Neurotransmitter	Purpose
Tyrosine	Folic acid, vitamins B3, B6, and Calcium, Copper	Dopamine, epinephrine, norepinephrine	Natural energizer, focus and concentration, addictions, cravings
Taurine, Glycine	Zinc, Manganese, Calcium, Magnesium	Gama-Aminobutyric Acid (GABA)	Natural sedative
Phenylalanine	Vitamins B6, B3, and Iron	Endorphins	Natural pain killer and pleasure provider
Tryptophan and 5HTP	Vitamin B6, Calcium, Essential Fatty Acids, Magnesium	Serotonin	Mood stabilizer, sleep promoter, calms central nervous system
Glutamine	Vitamin B6, Essential Fatty Acids	GABA	Mental ability, digestive tract health, helps clear ammonia especially from brain

Essential Fatty Acids

Eating the right kinds of fats is not only part of a successful recovery package from depression, anxiety, and fatigue, but is absolutely critical to life. A lipid (fat) membrane surrounds every cell in the body. Essential fatty acids (EFAs) are a vital component of these membranes, allowing cells to absorb the proper nutrients,

Eating the right kinds of fats is not only part of a successful recovery package from depression, anxiety, and fatigue, but is absolutely critical to life.

eliminate toxins, and generate energy. EFAs also support white blood cells of the immune system, which detect and destroy invading organisms.

Two essential fatty acids, which must come from a food source or in supplemental form, are Linoleic Acid and Alpha-Linolenic Acid. EFAs enable proper release of neurotransmitters, molecules that transfer signals between nerve cells. Every intricacy of these neuron-firing electrical signals is vital to not only the central nervous system but the digestive system, as well. Plus, the dry weight of the brain consists of sixty percent lipid (fatty) tissue, providing insulation for the nerve fibers. Fatty acids are crucial molecules that ensure the brain's integrity and ability to perform.

The body also requires polyunsaturated fatty acids (PUFA), essential fatty acids known as Omega 3 and Omega 6. Once again, they are called essential because they must come from a dietary food source or in supplemental form. Omega 3 is found in fish, flaxseed, evening primrose, borage, and black currant seed oils. Flaxseed oil is the world's richest source of Omega 3. At fifty-eight percent by weight, it contains over twice the amount as fish oils. However—and a big however—the body must undergo another metabolic process to convert flaxseed oil into Omega 3. Some individuals are unable to accomplish this conversion step due to ill health or other nutrient depletion.

Deep water, wild caught ocean fish such as salmon, tuna, mackerel, herring, and sardine are excellent, immediate sources of this alpha-linolenic Omega 3 fatty acid. This PUFA is also found in other vegetable seeds and nuts and their oils—such as hemp, chia, walnut, and pumpkin. The PUFA linoleic fatty acid, Omega 6, is most commonly found in raw and unheated safflower, sunflower, and sesame seeds and their oils.

Essential fatty acids attract oxygen and thereby operate as a biological equivalent of aspirin, providing some short term relief to arthritic symptoms. They can also enhance calcium absorption, and EFAs are very important for weight loss. They are nutrient dense and restore proper cellular function, eliminating cellular hunger and cravings. Eating the right kind of fat is key for weight loss, weight maintenance, and alleviating fatigue, depression, and anxiety. EFAs help premenstrual syndrome, attention deficit and hyperactivity disorder, multiple sclerosis (nerve transmission), intestinal health, skin, cardiovascular function, allergies, and hormone synthesis.

Essential fatty acids help to balance out all fatty acids, especially arachidonic acid. This necessary nutrient can reach toxic form with a diet high in corn-fed beef or any food that is excessively char-broiled or char-grilled. It is critical to balance all fatty acids in the body by adding the Omega 3 and Omega 6 PUFAs. Research shows that deficiencies of these EFAs are implicated in many neuropsychiatric diseases, including depression, anxiety, bipolar disorder, schizophrenia, Alzheimer's, and Parkinson's. Even DHA (docosahexaenoic acid), a component of Omega 3, unbalanced with EPA (eicosapentaenoic acid), also a component of Omega 3, was identified as a risk factor for anxiety disorders and post-partum depression.

Chart of Essential Fatty Acids

Essential Nutrients	Signs of Deficiency	Prevents Absorption	Supports Absorption	Food Sources
Linoleic and Linolenic Acids (Omega 3 and 6 PUFAs)	Dandruff, acne, dry skin and hair, fatigue, mental deterioration, immune depletion, inflammation	Radiation	Vitamins C, D, E, B-complex, choline, and calcium, zinc	Flaxseed oil and ground flaxseed, olive oil, borage oil, evening primrose oil, black currant oil

Studies on oconut oil have revealed its positive effects in preventing amyloid plaque formation by increasing antioxidant levels in the brain—very important research in Alzheimer's and other brain amyloid plaque diseases.

No discussion of healthy fats for balancing mental, emotional, and physical health would be complete without mentioning coconut oil. This amazing saturated fat—we need saturated fats, too—consists largely of medium-chain-triglycerides, which do not deposit in the fat cells like typical saturated fats, but is burned up relatively quickly. Scientific evaluation has proven the medicinal value of this wonderful healthy fat for its positive effects in relief from stress, anxiety, and depression. The complex lauric, capric, and caprylic components of this fatty acid have exhibited antibacterial and antifungal properties, and thus, is beneficial for gastrointestinal health. Studies on coconut oil have revealed its positive effects in preventing amyloid plaque formation by increasing antioxidant levels in the brain—very important research in Alzheimer's and other brain amyloid plaque diseases.

General Recommendations for Bloodwork and other Testing Guidelines

General blood work at a local lab is a good start. However, it will not detect a functional (precursor process) disease—only a disease that has already manifested itself. Moreover, general blood work results can be quite misleading relative to nutritional status—even cancer patients have reported perfect blood work. General blood work usually consists of a Complete Metabolic Panel (CMP) and a Complete Blood Count (CBC). They are routinely ordered, for instance, when you are admitted to the emergency room with overwhelming and critical symptoms.

The blood provides information about organ dysfunction, but does not reveal the basis for its dysfunction. In other words, from a routine blood test the presence of liver disease may be established, but identifying the root cause becomes another issue. Because a blood test doesn't disclose deficiency or toxicity, it is of little value in terms of designing a nutritional program.

Think of general blood work (or one single test, for that matter) as peering into only one window of a home you've never entered. A more complete picture of the functional layout of the home comes into view when you look into a few more windows or open a door or two. So it is with testing or screening—looking at the function of the body from many different angles with an eye to root cause—is critical to identifying and creating a path to optimal health.

Other nutritional screenings such as those listed below can serve as early warnings to prevent disease and take a more proactive approach to ideal health. Wisdom from God's Word in Jeremiah 31:21a instructs that we should, "Set up for yourself road marks, place for yourself guideposts; direct your mind to the highway, the way by which you went."

CMP Comprehensive Metabolic Panel—used as a broad screening tool to evaluate organ function and check for conditions such as diabetes, liver disease, and kidney disease already in progress.

CBC Complete Blood Count—measures various aspects of red and white blood cells including hemoglobin and hematocrit, which can point to anemia as well as potential viral, bacterial, and parasitic infections. Drink plenty of purified water prior to this test to rule out dehydration.

Following are other blood tests that I recommend as a more proactive approach and to determine baseline health. These tests can identify a potential functional disease already in progress so that nutritional programs and can stop or reverse the disease:

Ferritin—the ideal test to identify back-up iron stores. Low levels are always related to fatigue. High levels, known as hemochromatosis, are dangerous and not uncommon in men.

Hemoglobin A1C—three-month window to analyze how your body is processing blood sugar—a marker for diabetes risk or diagnosis.

Magnesium-RBC—measures red blood cell (not serum) stored levels of magnesium, which is necessary for most metabolic activity in the body. A marker for anxiety, depression, fatigue, and gut health.

Homocysteine—an amino acid produced by the body during the liver's methylation cycle. Elevated homocysteine is associated with many cardiovascular disorders such as increased risk of atherosclerosis, stroke, and abdominal aortic aneurysm. Elevation is usually due to deficiencies of Vitamin B12, Vitamin B6, and Folate. Other associated conditions are depression, anxiety, and fatigue.

Cardiac CRP (also known as HS CRP)—identifies inflammation, specifically cardiovascular. Studies have proven this marker far better than cholesterol in predicting cardiovascular events such as stroke and heart attack.

Vitamin B12—an energy marker critical to many biochemical pathways including the liver methylation pathway. Anyone on an acid-blocker, experiencing reflux or heartburn, or feeling a general sense of fatigue should get this test.

Methylmalonate (MMA)—a serum marker, which, if elevated, is an early indicator of vitamin B12 deficiency and implicated in many neurodegenerative diseases

Thyroid stimulating hormone (TSH)—this hormone is produced by the pituitary, which also produces the enzymes thyroid peroxidase (TPO), thyroglobulin (TG).

Free T3 and Free T4 thyroid hormones—T4 is converted to T3 in the liver and intestines, but only if there is enough healthy gut bacteria and the minerals iodine and selenium.

Reverse T3 thyroid hormone (rT3)—twenty percent of T4 becomes rT3 which is inactive. Reverse T3 becomes elevated during emotional or physical trauma, surgery, or chronic illness.

Thyroid Peroxidase (TPO) and Thyroglobulin (TG) Antibodies—measures antibodies produced by the immune system against the thyroid hormones, indicating Hashimoto's thyroiditis autoimmune disease.

Vitamin D-25-Hydroxy—an excellent marker for inflammation. Adequate levels are important to prevent of all kinds of inflammatory diseases including depression and colon cancer, and hormonally related cancers of the breast, prostate, and uterus. This vitamin, which is sometimes referred to as a hormone in the research, is important for essential bone building, cardiovascular, neuromuscular, and brain health, as well as prevention of gastrointestinal diseases and Alzheimer's and Parkinson's.

I also recommend the following non-traditional health panels, which have further potential to identify a functional disease process, so that steps may be taken to reverse the progress:

Adrenal Cortisol Panel—measures four salivary cortisol levels throughout the day. This information is significant to evaluate energy production, as well as anxiety and depression.

Methyltetrahydrofolate-reductase (MTHF-R)—cheek swab or blood test that identifies faulty gene or polymorphism for this enzyme, which converts folic acid to its activated, usable form, 5-MTHF.

Catechol-o-methyl transferase (COMT)—cheek swab that identifies faulty gene for this enzyme, which is involved in neurotransmitter conversion.

In my clinical experience, over ninety-percent of patients show signs of zinc deficiency.

Zinc Taste Test (ZTT)—in office test instantly determines your zinc status. Zinc is a co-factor for almost every biochemical function that takes place. Gustin is the major zinc protein found in the saliva of the parotid gland. If zinc status is sufficient, then the immediate reaction to a small dose of liquid zinc sulfate is a metallic taste. If zinc is insufficient, the dose will taste like water. In my clinical experience, over ninety-percent of patients show signs of zinc deficiency.

Gastrointestinal Health Panel—tests for digestion and absorption of protein, fat and carbohydrates, as well as inflammatory markers, including yeast/fungus and bacteria.

Hair Mineral Analysis—hair tissue sample indicates levels of twelve critical minerals, plus heavy metals that include lead, cadmium, arsenic, mercury, and aluminum. Levels of these minerals and metals identify organ, gland, and body system imbalances, including mental and emotional.

Hormone Panel—salivary test for estradiol, estrone, estriol, progesterone, 17-OH-progesterone, testosterone, and DHEA. Studies have shown saliva tests for actually available hormones to be more accurate than blood tests.

Gluten Sensitivity Test—saliva test for antibodies produced by the immune system against gliadin, a protein found in gluten, which determines your sensitivity to wheat, rye, barley, and other gluten-containing grains.

Neurotransmitter Panel—urine collection for serotonin, dopamine, GABA, glutamate, PEA, epinephrine, and norepinephrine. When unbalanced, these chemical messengers can result in anxiety, depression, insomnia, ADD, OCD, fatigue, cravings, and eating disorders.

Organic Acids Test—measures urinary markers for organic acids in the form of end-metabolites, which indicate arabinose (the marker for candida), and eight other yeast/fungus markers. This test also exposes markers including bacteria such as clostridia, as well as oxalates, mitochondrial (energy) function, neurotransmitters, B vitamins, vitamin C, CoQ10, and others.

GPL-Tox Screen—measures eighteen different metabolites, which are urinary markers for over one-hundred-seventy different environmental pollutants, such as phthalates, pesticides, and organophosphates.

SIBO Test—breath test (yes, you send your breath off to the lab) that measures hydrogen and methane gas produced by the small intestine, which are markers for small intestinal bacterial overgrowth.

Hpylori Test—the gold-standard breath test that measures hydrogen gas produced by Hpylori bacteria in the stomach.

Food Allergy/Sensitivity Panels—laboratory finger-prick blood spot test identifies IgG antibodies to over seventy-five foods which determine delayed food allergy reactions that can occur within a seventy-two hour period after ingesting a particular food.

Chemstrip Urine Test—in-office test measures thirteen separate urine categories for infections, tissue degeneration, liver disease, kidney disease, and diabetes.

Conclusion

"Blessed is the man who trusts in the LORD, and whose trust is the LORD. For he will be like a tree planted by the water, that extends its roots by a stream, and will not fear when the heat comes; but its leaves will be green, and it will not be anxious in a year of drought nor cease to yield fruit."

Jeremiah 17:7-8

Hope for Healing

Clients rarely visit my office for the specific goal of weight loss. By the time they decide to see me they know that excess weight is not the problem, but a symptom of deeper biochemical issues. Hope is available, no matter what your current state of health. If you aren't feeling well, perhaps you should consult a medical doctor. But medical doctors may not have all the answers. Many physicians are prejudiced by the diagnosis. In other words, many diagnosed illnesses or diseases have a pre-conceived medical route, which in most cases utilizes pharmaceutical drugs as the only option. Many physicians follow conventional drug protocols without digging deeper to find and unload root causes.

Don't lose your identity because of physical or emotional pain or any kind of diagnosis. Our society seems to promote a 'victim' mentality. If you don't feel well you should seek an appropriate diagnosis. But a diagnosis does not excuse personal responsibility, nor pronounce you a victim.

Victimhood disempowers a person—I call this wilderness thinking. The Israelites turned what should have been an eleven-day journey into forty years wandering in the wilderness. Fear, rejection, shame, and guilt create a vicious cycle if you stay steeped in victimhood, which is exactly what the enemy of your soul wants. Do you have wilderness thinking? If you have compassionate honesty regarding your particular diagnosis, then you can release

You are no longer a victim with a victim mentality; you are an overcomer because you have victory through Jesus Christ.

the bondage that the disease and the enemy might otherwise claim. Your mind is now free to realize all the available choices—to create hope and to heal both physically and emotionally. You are no longer a victim with a victim mentality; you are an overcomer because you have victory through Jesus Christ.

> *I have been crucified with Christ; and it is no longer I who live, but Christ lives in me, and the life which I now live in the flesh I live by faith in the Son of God, who loved me and gave Himself up for me.*
>
> Galatians 2:20

Take responsibility to educate yourself about your doctor's course of treatment and other alternatives. Each one of us must gather sufficient information about maintaining a healthy body. If confusion sets in because of the wide variety of conflicting suggestions and wacky information on the internet, then ask the Holy Spirit to lead you to a root-cause health care provider whom you can trust. Wise choices are the fruit of knowledge. Hosea 4:6 says, "My people are destroyed for lack of knowledge." Your body can reverse the course of long-term illness and disease with wise choices.

Now the decision to seek optimal health, regardless of your diagnosis, rests with you. Do you believe that God can heal you physically and emotionally? Healing is available to you, just like it was to the Capernaum woman in the gospel of Mark. She believed that if she could only touch the hem of Jesus' garment then she would be healed. She did and she was.

> *And a woman who had a hemorrhage for twelve years, and had endured much at the hands of many physicians, and had spent all that she had and was not helped at all, but rather had*

> *grown worse, after hearing about Jesus, came up in the crowd behind Him, and touched His cloak. For she thought, "If I just touch His garments, I shall get well." And immediately the flow of her blood was dried up; and she felt in her body that she was healed of her affliction.*
>
> Mark 5:25-29

Grab the hem of His garment, oh precious child of God! God can miraculously heal you in an instant, like He did this woman from Capernaum, or He may choose to heal you over time. Without faith, there is no hope. Not faith in a health care practitioner or a physician or a drug or a supplement, but faith in the One God who created your entire being, your chemistry lab. No one knows your body better than you do, except Him. You can choose to take responsibility for the health of your beautiful body and mind. Then, and only then, will you be motivated to move forward, creating hope through God-appointed self-healing.

Prepare ahead of time. First Peter 1:13 instructs:

> *Therefore, prepare your minds for action, keep sober in spirit, fix your hope completely on the grace to be brought to you at the revelation of Jesus Christ.*

Ask the Holy Spirit to intervene and bring your flesh under His control. Repeat your petition over and over until it becomes a fleshly and a spiritual habit. You must plan (or have someone help you plan) your way, and He will direct your steps. He will make known to you the path of life; you will find complete joy and pleasure in His presence as you walk the path with Him. The God of Israel will go before you and He will be your rear guard.

> *The mind of man plans his way, but the LORD directs his steps.*
>
> Proverbs 16:9

You will make known to me the path of life; in Your presence is fullness of joy; in Your right hand there are pleasures forever.

Psalm 16:11

For the Lord will go before you, and the God of Israel will be your rear guard.

Isaiah 52:12b

Oh dear, precious saint, His Word holds so many promises—none of us should ever experience a moment of anxiety, depression, or fatigue as we follow the path He has laid out for us. However, the Bible tells us about some saints who God called specifically to carry out His instructions, and who experienced the same human frailties as you and me. Elijah is a good example—a man God appointed who was following His path, but ran in fear from Jezebel, and sunk into depression under a juniper tree in the wilderness, and asked God to take his life. However, God revived Elijah through an extended time of rest, sleep, water, and food provided by an angel. He got up rested and refreshed, ready to take responsibility and obey God. We, too, should be in relentless pursuit of who God made us to be.

God called me to be an ambassador and proclaim all that He has done for me in His constant faithfulness. In Jeremiah 31:3-4, His promise to you and me is:

I have loved you with an everlasting love; therefore I have drawn you with lovingkindness. Again I will build you, and you shall be rebuilt.

Lovingkindness is perhaps one of my favorite words in the Bible. I have always regarded it as symbolic, illuminating, and lengthy—the word goes on and on and on, just like His love, grace, and mercy. He peels, reveals, and heals, if you will allow Him.

Finally, if you don't know the God Who created you or His Son, Jesus, or the power of God that comes from His Holy Spirit residing in you, there is a way you can have that peace which surpasses all human understanding. Not a limited, human peace, but an unyielding peace. Recognize and accept that God came to earth in human form as the Man, Jesus, over two-thousand years ago. He came so that we might have eternal life starting now, with an eternally pure and perfect body to come.

In John 14:6, Jesus said, "I am the way, and the truth, and the life; no one comes to the Father but through Me." Jesus is the bridge over an eternal gap, a gap between us and a holy God, created by our sin. Jesus died a horrible death through crucifixion as resolution of all sin for those who believe. Then, after three days, He defeated death and arose from the grave fully alive, just as He said He would. He ascended to heaven and assigned the Holy Spirit of God as our counselor, our comforter, and our friend.

I love the song "Already There," by *Casting Crowns.* Some of the amazing lyrics are:

"One day I'll stand before You
and look back on the life I've lived
'cause You're already there,
You're already there.
When I'm lost in the mystery,
to You my future is a memory
'cause You're already there."

That surely gives me great peace, and I hope it does you, too, because He knows it ALL!

My Own Journey: The Author's Journey to Wholeness and Wellness

My path to physical healing was littered with emotional scarring from spiritual roots of childhood abuse. At a very young age, I discovered protection through dissociation by emotionally stepping outside my body during sexual abuse. I found other creative ways to deal with similarly destructive situations. I realized the powerful comfort and safety of food—another subconscious self-preservation mechanism to make myself undesirable to my abuser. Unknown to me at the time, food also helped bury the pain, shame, and guilt. The trauma set the stage for decades of unbalanced physical, emotional, and spiritual health.

My mother died of melanoma on my seventeenth birthday. As the second oldest of eleven children, I became the surrogate mother for three years preceding her death onward. Not only had I kept my "baby fat", by the time I graduated from high school, I weighed two-hundred-eleven pounds. I then determined to be thin and lost a total of sixty pounds over the next one-and-one-half years. I thought I had triumphed in all my battles.

But my subconscious self-preservation mechanisms continued to operate in all areas of my life until my late thirties. I noticed a recurrent pattern of emotionally and potentially physically harmful relationships repeating themselves in my life. My best friend at the time suggested that I try psychological counseling. But I didn't see any need for it. I'd always been able to handle everything else in my life by myself; I should be able to handle this as well.

Fork in the Road

In 1989, when I was thirty-eight, I reached a fork in the road of my life. It was a pivotal time when I would choose the road that would carry me on my journey to physical and emotional healing and spiritual salvation. By this time, I had been working full time since I was seventeen. I had earned degrees in Cosmetology and Business, birthed and reared a child, married and divorced, and was climbing the proverbial corporate ladder. I thought I had all that I could want, yet I was desperately unhappy.

At that time I had been in the corporate field for eighteen years. I was a product sales manager for a large industrial manufacturer traveling extensively in the United States, Mexico, Canada, and Europe. As a type A personality, an introvert with a predominately melancholy personality, I was making as much money as I had ever made in my life. I excelled as a female salesperson in a male dominated industry. I loved the positive recognition from men—something I never received as a child. But anyone who has worked in the corporate arena knows that more is never enough. Goals are always set higher, and achievement is expected. I was driven to be the best and to accomplish the most in the shortest amount of time.

From all external appearances, I should have been happy. I was a single mother of a well-adjusted, good boy who had just turned a teenager. I had lots of friends, a wonderful bunch of brothers and sisters, a nice car, a lovely home, and a great job. I wondered why I was so desperately unhappy and why I felt such emptiness in my life. I had unwittingly traveled down a path of innocent and naive self-destruction, both physically and emotionally.

Self-Destruction or Salvation

Then God began to reveal things to me. I remember clearly reading an Ann Landers article describing a young woman sexually abused by her father, and I began thinking about the pain and disgust of incest. A hint of the possibility of similar abuse in my own life flashed over me. I immediately dismissed it engaging the denial mechanism, telling myself that no father could do such an abominable thing to a daughter.

But the notion persisted and finally drove me to counseling for major depression and to unravel the destructive pattern in my life—seeking relationships with men who were unavailable physically and emotionally. I learned that I was only repeating what I experienced as a child and teenager. In 1990, through very intensive psychotherapy, I realized I was suffering from post-traumatic stress disorder and began to acknowledge the trauma I suffered as the victim of childhood abuse.

I carried on with my job the best I could, experiencing unimaginable random flashbacks at totally unexpected times. The combined stressors of extensive business traveling, the maternal guilt for leaving my son, and overwhelming childhood traumas of recollected repressed memories was more than my body could bear. I began to experience symptoms ranging from incredible fatigue and exhaustion to severe abdominal cramping. I could not form a complete thought pattern. I could not place one word in front of another to form a complete sentence. I desperately tried to cover-up the depression and exhaustion with a smiling face and clever make-up. But deception exacerbated the exhaustion. The lie continued for a little while longer. Eventually, I could no longer cover the grayish complexion and the hollow, empty eyes that held no sparkle.

At the same time that my emotional and physical issues were surfacing, I accepted Jesus as Lord and Savior of my life. Although I had found a bright spot in my life, things got progressively worse. But He is faithful! I consulted with many doctors, but none could tell me what was wrong with me because all my blood work was perfect. Each was eager to prescribe an antidepressant. But I believed more was involved than depression—I had to find the root cause for all my distress.

Diagnosis at Last

After more than a year, I finally found a medical doctor who believed strongly that nutrition is a critical basis for good health. Yes, a medical doctor! I was diagnosed with thirteen different "diseases" that manifested an endless number of symptoms: diverticulosis, hypothyroidism, hypoglycemia, hypoadrenal, PMS, malfunctioning liver, mitral valve prolapse, systemic fungal disease (candida), post-traumatic stress disorder, hormonal imbalances, chronic fatigue, major depression, and the early stages of gallstones.

These were the physiological symptoms of the incredible depression. I began to despair. The sicker I became physically, the sicker I became emotionally—or was it the other way around? I did not want to live; I did not want to "be." I felt like I was being literally twisted inside. Perhaps, if I twisted hard enough, I could make myself disappear. I cannot adequately describe the agony of being inside myself, or the agony of being around people, or talking to anyone, even my best friend. I was paralyzed with guilt and shame without knowing why. But I found a Christian counselor who helped me get to the root of my spiritual bondage.

God's Plan

As much as I hurt emotionally and physically, I knew God had a plan for me. Genesis 41:51 and 52 were prophetic words from women of God who prayed over me. "... God has made me forget all my trouble and all my father's household, and ... God has made me fruitful in the land of my affliction."

I hung onto His promises. As I became healthier physically, emotionally, and spiritually through nutritional and emotional counseling, I knew what the Lord was calling me to do. But He only revealed His plan to me one day at a time. Proverbs 16:9 repeated over and over in my mind: "The mind of man plans his way, but the Lord directs his steps."

With the powerful trust of a new Christian, I quit my almost six-figure income job and launched my education in nutrition and the natural health sciences. The Lord once again spoke to me through Isaiah 61:1: "The spirit of the Lord God is upon me because the Lord has anointed me to bring good news to the afflicted. He has sent me to bind up the brokenhearted."

Forgiveness Provides a Deeper and Locked-In Healing

As I continued through the process of healing, I learned the great power of forgiveness. Only by the power of His Holy Spirit in me have I been able to forgive both my father and my mother—my father for the abuse and my mother for not protecting me. What a powerful release I experienced through that forgiveness! The shame and guilt I carried all my life belonged to my perpetrators, and the forgiveness allowed me to release those heavy burdens.

There is still that little girl inside me who wants to wave her magic wand and make the whole world right and clean and new. But now I realize that no magic wand and no magic pill exists. I am not responsible for the whole world; I am responsible for myself and to God. Understanding, healing, and growth come through courage, willingness, determination, discipline, and the pain of change. The reward then becomes the opportunity to pluck the fruit of wise choices. I would not be writing this book if I had not taken personal responsibility to recover my health. I would be blessed to know that the information presented in this book has helped you or a loved one in exchanging fear for hope, and pain for joy as you experience God-ordained healing.

References

Introduction

Albert, P. "Why is depression more prevalent in women?" *J Psychiatry Neurosci*, 2015 Jul.

Cyranowski, J., et al. "Adolescent onset of the gender difference in lifetime rates of major depression: a theoretical model." *Arch Gen Psychiatry*, 2000 Jan.

Burton, Neel. "The 7 Reasons Why Depression is more Common in Women." Psychology Today. https://www.psychologytoday.com/blog/hide-and-seek/201205/the-7-reasons-why-depression-is-more-common-in-women.

Part One – Health the Way God Intended

Chambers, Oswald. *My Utmost for His Highest.* Grand Rapids: Discovery House Publishers, 1992.

Mendelsohn, Robert. *Mal(e) Practice: How Doctors Manipulate Women.* Chicago: Contemporary Books, 1982.

Brand, Paul, Paul Yancy. *In His Image.* Grand Rapids: Zondervan, 1984.

Part Two – Your Divine Chemistry Lab

Fröhlich, E., et al. "Cognitive impairment by antibiotic-induced gut dysbiosis: Analysis of gut microbiota-brain communication." *Brain Behav Immun*, 2016 Feb.

Paul, B., et al. "Influences of diet and the gut microbiome on epigenetic modulation in cancer and other diseases." *Clin Epigenetics*, 2015 Oct.

Mercola, Joseph. "Your Genes Remember a Sugar Hit." http://articles.mercola.com/sites/articles/archive/2009/02/12/your-genes-remember-a-sugar-hit.aspx.

Weinhold, B. "Epigenetics: The Science of Change." *Environ Health Perspect*, 2006 March.

Fenech, M., et al. "The effect of age, gender, diet and lifestyle on DNA damage measured using micronucleus frequency in human peripheral blood lymphocytes." Oxford University Press on behalf of the UK Environmental Mutagen Society, 2010 August.

Akdogan, R., et al. "A pilot study of Helicobacter pylori genotypes and cytokine gene polymorphisms in reflux oesophagitis and peptic ulcer disease." *Bratisl Lek Listy*, 2014.

Mowat, A., et al. "Regional specialization within the intestinal immune system." *Nat Rev Immunol*, 2014 Oct.

Jurgelewicz, M. "Assessing and Supporting Methylation Pathways." *Designs for Health*, 2015 Feb.

Schafer, J., et al. "Homocysteine and Cognitive Function in a Population-based Study of Older Adults." *J Am Geriatr Soc*, 2005.

Rudenko, A., et al. "Epigenetic modifications in the nervous system and their impact upon cognitive impairments." *Neuropharmacology*, 2013 May.

Levin, J., et al. "Elevated levels of methylmalonate and homocysteine in

Parkinson's disease, progressive supranuclear palsy and amyotrophic lateral sclerosis." *Dement Geriatr Cogn Disord*, 2010.

Pizzorno, Joseph E., Michael T. Murray. "Detoxification: A Naturopathic Perspective." *Natural Medicine Journal*, May 1998.

Haenisch, B., et.al. "Risk of dementia in elderly patients with the use of proton pump inhibitors." *European Archives of Psychiatry & Clinical Neuroscience*, Aug 2015.

Whittekin, Martie. *Natural Alternatives to Nexium, Maalox, Tagamet, Prilosec & other Acid Blockers.* Garden City Park, NY: Square One Publishers, 2009.

Lam, J., et al. "Proton pump inhibitor and histamine 2 receptor antagonist use and vitamin B12 deficiency." *JAMA*, 2013 Dec.

Jackson, M., et al. "Proton pump inhibitors alter the composition of the gut microbiota." *Gut*, 2015 Dec.

Gomm, W., et al. "Association of Proton Pump Inhibitors With Risk of Dementia: A Pharmacoepidemiological Claims Data Analysis." *JAMA Neurol.*, 2016 Feb.

Braun-Moscovici, Y., et al. "What tests should you use to assess small intestinal bacterial overgrowth in systemic sclerosis?" *Clin Exp Rheumatol*, 2015 Jul-Aug.

Miazga, A., et al. "Current views on the etiopathogenesis, clinical manifestation, diagnostics, treatment and correlation with other nosological entities of SIBO." *Adv Med Sci*, 2015 Mar.

Thibodeau, Gary, Kevin Patton. *The Human Body in Health & Disease*. St. Louis: Mosby-Year Book, Inc., 2002

Part Three – What Causes a Toxic Body?

Ulluwishewa, D., et al. "Regulation of Tight Junction Permeability by Intestinal Bacteria and Dietary Components." *The Journal of Nutrition*, 2011 Mar.

Fasano, A., "Leaky gut and autoimmune diseases." *Clin Rev Allergy Immunol*, 2012 Feb.

Fasano, A. "Zonulin and Its Regulation of Intestinal Barrier Function: The Biological Door to Inflammation, Autoimmunity, and Cancer." *Physiological Reviews*, 2011 Jan.

Fasano, A. "Zonulin, regulation of tight junctions, and autoimmune diseases." Ann N Y Acad Sci, 2012 Jul.

Drago, S., et al. "Gliadin, zonulin and gut permeability: Effects on celiac and non-celiac intestinal mucosa and intestinal cell lines." *Scand J Gastroenterol*, 2006 Apr.

Sapone, A., et al. "Zonulin Upregulation Is Associated With Increased Gut Permeability in Subjects With Type 1 Diabetes and Their Relatives." *Diabetes*, 2006 May vol. 55.

Odenwald, M., et al. "Intestinal permeability defects: is it time to treat?" *Clin Gastroenterol Hepato*l, 2013 Sept.

Liu, Z., et al. "Tight junctions, leaky intestines, and pediatric diseases." *Acta Paediatr*, 2005 April.

Owczarek, D., et al. "Diet and nutritional factors in inflammatory bowel diseases." *World J Gastroenterol*, 2016 Jan.

Santelmann, H., Howard, J. "Yeast metabolic products, yeast antigens and yeasts as possible triggers for irritable bowel syndrome." *Eur J Gastroenterol Hepatol*, 2005 Jan.

Bakri, M., et al. "In vitro expression of Candida albicans alcohol dehydrogenase genes involved in acetaldehyde metabolism." *Mol Oral Microbiol*, 2015 Feb.

Uittamo, J., et al. "Xylitol inhibits carcinogenic acetaldehyde production by Candida species." *Int J Cancer*, 2011 Oct.

Kaufmann, Doug. *The Fungus Link to Health Problems*. Rockwall: MediaTrition; Third Edition 2010.

Lopez, D, et al. "Biofilms." *Cold Spring Harb Perspect Biol*, 2010 Jul.

Bjarnsholt, T. "The role of bacterial biofilms in chronic infections." APMIS Suppl, 2013 May.

Wolcott, R., Ehrlich, G. "Biofilms and chronic infections." *JAMA*, 2008 June.

Lee, H., et al. "Synergistic inhibition of streptococcal biofilm by ribose and xylitol." *Arch Oral Biol*, 2015 Feb.

Olmstead, Stephen. Biofilms part 1: the mycobiome, candida, and gastrointestinal health. *ProThera, Inc. Practitioner Newsletter*, Feb 2016.

Packiavathy, I., et al. "Inhibition of biofilm development of uropathogens by curcumin—an antiquorum sensing agent from Curcuma longa." *Food Chem*, 2014 April.

Shahzad, M., et al. "Utilising polyphenols for the clinical management of Candida albicans biofilms." *Int J Antimicrob Agents*, 2014 Sept.

Dovigo, L., et al. "Susceptibility of clinical isolates of Candida to photodynamic effects of curcumin." *Lasers Surg Med*, 2011 Nov.

Yang, F., et al. "Curcumin inhibits formation of amyloid beta oligomers and fibrils, binds plaques, and reduces amyloid in vivo." *J Biol Chem*, Feb2005.

Kondo, K., et al. "Identification of a novel HHV-6 latent-protein associated with CFS and mood disorders." The Jikei University School of Medicine, Tokyo. *Symposia Brain Science on Fatigue: New Insights from Viral Reactivation, Cytokines and Imaging*, 2010 Dec.

Tlaskalová-Hogenová, H., et al. "Commensal bacteria (normal microflora), mucosal immunity and chronic inflammatory and autoimmune diseases." *Immunol Lett*, 2004 Ma.y

Sharma, P., et al. "Effect of Yoga-Based Intervention in Patients with Inflammatory Bowel Disease." *Int J Yoga Therap*, 2015.

Wouters, M., et al. "Is there a causal link between psychological disorders and functional gastrointestinal disorders?" *Expert Rev Gastroenterol Hepatol*, 2016 Jan.

Part Four – Anxiety & Depression are Not All in Your Head

Sapolsky, Robert. *Why Zebras Don't Get Ulcers*. New York: WH Freeman and Company, 1994.

Price, Sharon R. *The Pathophysiology of Stress, Adrenal Activity, and the Causal Chain of Body Weight Dysfunction in Women*. Birmingham: PhD Natural

Health Science, 2002.
Du, J., et al. "The Role of Nutrients in Protecting Mitochondrial Function and Neurotransmitter Signaling: Implications for the Treatment of Depression, PTSD, and Suicidal Behaviors." *Crit Rev Food Sci Nutr*, 2014 Nov.
Roy, A., et al. "Monoamines, glucose metabolism, aggression towards self and others." *Int J Neurosci*, 1988 Aug.
Andradea, M., et al. "A Reexamination of the Hypoglycemia Aggression Hypothesis in Laboratory Mice." International *Journal of Neuroscience*, Volume 41, Issue 3-4, 1988.
Schoenthaler, S., et al. "Applied Nutrition and Behavior." International Academy of Nutrition and Preventive Medicine, *Journal of Applied Nutrition*, Vol 43 No 1, 1991.
Eastern Kentucky University. "Human Physiology-Neurons & the Nervous System BIO 301" http://people.eku.edu/ritchisong/301notes2.htm.
Yano, J., et al. "Indigenous Bacteria from the Gut Microbiota Regulate Host Serotonin Biosynthesis." http://resolver.caltech.edu/CaltechAUTHORS:20150409-093248232.
Szabo, S., Tache, Y. "The legacy of Hans Selye and the origins of stress research: A retrospective 75 years after his landmark brief." Letter to the Editor of Nature Stress, 2012 September
Stokes, P. "The potential role of excessive cortisol induced by HPA hyperfunction in the pathogenesis of depression." European *Neuropsychopharmacology*, 1995.
Wilson, James. *Adrenal Fatigue-the 21st Century Stress Syndrome.* Petaluma: Smart Publications, 2001.
Nevlan, T., et al. "Cortisol levels predict cognitive impairment induced by electroconvulsive therapy." *Biol Psychiatry*, 2001 Sep.
The Jason Foundation. "Youth Suicide Statistics." http://jasonfoundation.com/prp/facts/youth-suicide-statistics/.
Adolescent and School Health. "Youth Risk Behavior Surveillance System (YRBSS)." http://www.cdc.gov/healthyyouth/data/yrbs/index.htm.
American Association for Marriage and Family Therapy. "Post-Traumatic Stress Disorder." http://www.aamft.org/iMIS15/AAMFT/Content/consumer_updates/post-traumatic_stress_disorder.aspx.
Schmidt, A., Thews, G. "Autonomic Nervous System". I*n Janig, W. Human Physiology* (2 ed.). New York, NY: Springer-Verlag. pp. 333–370 1989.
Hart, Archibald. *The Hidden Link Between Adrenaline and Stress.* Dallas: Word Publishing, 1995.
Montero, G., et al. "Wilson disease: liver form." *Rev Gastroenterol* Peru, 2015 Oct-Dec.
Frieden, E., Hsieh, H. "Ceruloplasmin: the copper transport protein with essential oxidase activity." *Adv Enzymol Relat Areas Mol Biol*, 1976.
Evans, G., Wiederanders, R. "Pituitary-adrenal regulation of ceruloplasmin." *Nature* 1967 Aug.
Olsson, E., et al. "A randomised, double-blind, placebo-controlled, parallel-group study of the standardised extract shr-5 of the roots of Rhodiola rosea in the

treatment of subjects with stress-related fatigue." *Planta Med*, Feb 2009.

Hellhammer, J., et al. "Omega-3 fatty acids administered in phosphatidylserine improved certain aspects of high chronic stress in men." *Nutr Res*, 2012 April.

Black, C., et al. "Is depression associated with increased oxidative stress? A systematic review and meta-analysis." *Psychoneuroendocrinology*, 2015 Jan.

Part Five - The Inflammatory Role in Depression and Anxiety

Gershon, Michael. *The Second Brain*. New York: Harper Collins, 1998.

Baruk, H. "Experimental catatonia and the problem of will and personality." *J. Nerv Ment Dis*, 110, 218-234, 1949.

Sherwin, E., et al. "A gut (microbiome) feeling about the brain." *Curr Opin Gastroenterol*, 2016 Mar.

Kukla, U., et al. "Mental disorders in digestive system diseases - internist's and psychiatrist's insight." *Pol Merkur Lekarski*. 2015 May.

Evrensel, A., et al. "The Gut-Brain Axis: The Missing Link in Depression." *Clin Psychopharmacol Neurosci*, 2015 Dec .

Heyman, M., et al. "Cytokine-induced alteration of the epithelial barrier to food antigens in disease." *Ann N Y Acad Sci*, 2000.

Heuvelin, E., et al. "Mechanisms involved in alleviation of intestinal inflammation by bifidobacterium breve soluble factors." *PLoS One*, 2009.

Heyman, M., et al. "Mononuclear cells from infants allergic to cow's milk secrete tumor necrosis factor alpha, altering intestinal function." *Gastroenterology*, 1994 June.

Meeker, S., et al. "Protective links between vitamin D, inflammatory bowel disease and colon cancer." *World J Gastroenterol*, 2016 Jan.

Kurina, L., et al. "Depression and anxiety in people with inflammatory bowel disease." *J. Epidemiol Community Health*, 2001 October.

Turner, E., et al. "Selective publication of antidepressant trials and its influence on apparent efficacy." *N Engl J Med*, 2008 Jan.

Weissman, M., et al. "Offspring of Depressed Parents: 30 Years Later." Am J Psychiatry, 2016 Apr.

Wiley, J., et al. "Stress and glucocorticoid receptor transcriptional programming in time and space: Implications for the brain-gut axis." *Neurogastroenterol Moti*, 2016 Jan.

Kelly, J., et al. "Breaking down the barriers: the gut microbiome, intestinal permeability and stress-related psychiatric disorders." *Front Cell Neurosci*, 2015 Oct.

Nemani, K., et al. "Schizophrenia and the gut-brain axis." *Prog Neuropsychopharmacol Biol Psychiatry*,2015 Jan.

Burokas, A., et al. "Microbiota regulation of the Mammalian gut-brain axis." *Adv Appl Microbiol*, March 2015.

Cohen, S., et al. "Chronic stress, glucocorticoid receptor resistance, inflammation, and disease risk." *Proceedings of the National Academy of Sciences*, 2012 April 17.

Allison, D., et al. "The common inflammatory etiology of depression and cognitive impairment: a therapeutic target." *Journal of Neuroinflammation*, 2014 Sep.

Haroon, E. et al. "Psychoneuroimmunology meets neuropsychopharmacology: translational implications of the impact of inflammation on behavior." *Neuropsychopharmacology*, 2012 Jan.

Cohen, S., et al. "Chronic stress, glucocorticoid receptor resistance, inflammation, and disease risk." *Proc Natl Acad Sci U S A*. 2012 Apr.

O'Malley, D. "Immunomodulation of enteric neural function in irritable bowel syndrome." *World J Gastroenterol*, 2015 Jun.

Severance, E., et al. "Gastrointestinal inflammation and associated immune activation in schizophrenia." *Schizophr Res*, 2012 Jun.

Karakula-Juchnowicz, H., et al. "The role of IgG hypersensitivity in the pathogenesis and therapy of depressive disorders. " *Nutr Neurosci*, 2014 Sep.

Porcelli, B., et al. "Celiac and non-celiac gluten sensitivity: a review on the association with schizophrenia and mood disorders." *Auto Immun Highlights*, 2014 Oct.

Urban-Kowalczyk, M., et al. "Neuropsychiatric symptoms and celiac disease." *Neuropsychiatr Dis Treat*, 2014 Oct.

Cina, S., Perper, J. "Is lymphocytic (hashimoto) thyroiditis associated with suicide?" *Am J Forensic Med Pathol*, 2009 Sep.

Fam, J., et al. "Thyroid Autoimmune Antibodies and Major Depressive Disorder in Women." *Ann Acad Med Singapore*, 2015 Aug.

Bocchetta, A., et al. "Bipolar disorder and antithyroid antibodies: review and case series." *Int J Bipolar Disord*, 2016 Dec.

Krysiak, R., et al. "Sexual function and depressive symptoms in young women with thyroid autoimmunity and subclinical hypothyroidism." *Clin Endocrinol* (Oxf), 2016 Jun.

Giynas Ayhan, M., et al. "The prevalence of depression and anxiety disorders in patients with euthyroid Hashimoto's thyroiditis: a comparative study." *Gen Hosp Psychiatry*, 2014 Jan-Feb.

Kharrazian, Datis. *Why Do I Still Have Thyroid Symptoms? ...When My Lab Tests Are Normal.* Carlsbad: Elephant Press, 2010.

Vogelzangs, N., et al. "Cytokine production capacity in depression and anxiety." *Transl Psychiatry*, 2016 May.

Markus, J., et al. "Inflammation and Specific Symptoms of Depression." *JAMA Psychiatry*, 2016.

Zhu, M., et al. "Th1/Th2/Th17 cells imbalance in patients with asthma with and without psychological symptoms. *Allergy Asthma Proc*, 2016 Mar.

Lees, L., et al. "Cytokines in Neuropathic Pain and Associated Depression." *Mod Trends Pharmacopsychiatri*, 2015.

Goodhart, P., et al. "Mechanism-based inactivation of dopamine beta-hydroxylase by p-cresol and related alkylphenols." *Biochemistry*, 1987 May.

Part Six – Restoring Mental and Emotional Health through the Gut Highway

Ten Boom, Corrie. *The Hiding Place.* New Jersey: Fleming H. Revell Company, 1971.

U.S. Food and Drug Administration. "Polyethylene Glycol (PEG) 3350 over-the-counter oral laxative (Miralax), Potential Signals of Serious Risks/ New Safety Information Identified by the Adverse Event Reporting System (AERS) between October-December 2011" http://www.fda.gov/Drugs/GuidanceComplianceRegulatoryInformation/Surveillance/AdverseDrugEffects/ucm295585.htm.

National Institute for Occupational Safety and Health (NIOSH). "ETHYLENE GLYCOL:Systemic Agent." http://www.cdc.gov/niosh/ershdb/emergencyresponsecard_29750031.html.

Shirer, Priscilla. The Armor of God. Nashville: LifeWay Press, 2015

Black, C., et al. "Is depression associated with increased oxidative stress? A systematic review and met-analysis." *Psychoneuroendocrinology*, 2015 January.

Townsley, Cheryl. *Discovering Wholeness, the Spirit, Soul & Body Connection.* Littleton: LFH Publishing, 2000.

Morris, Robert. *The God I Never Knew.* Colorado Springs: Waterbrook Press, 2011.

Rogers, Sherry. *Tired or Toxic, a Blueprint for Health.* Syracuse: Prestige Publishers, 1990.

Schulte, E., et al. "Neural systems implicated in obesity as an addictive disorder: from biological to behavioral mechanisms." *Prog Brain Res*, 2015 Oct.

Lemieux, A., et al. "Stress psychobiology in the context of addiction medicine: from drugs of abuse to behavioral addictions." *Prog Brain Res*, 2015 Nov.

Moore, Beth. *Living Beyond Yourself.* Nashville: LifeWay Press, 1998.

Selhub, E., et al. "Fermented foods, microbiota, and mental health: ancient practice meets nutritional psychiatry." *Journal Physiol Anthropol*, 2014 Jan.

Abuajah, C., et al. "Functional components and medicinal properties of food: a review." J Food Sci Technol, 2015 May

Tamang, J., et al. "Functional Properties of Microorganisms in Fermented Foods." *Front Microbiol*, 2016 Apr.

Bourrie, B., et al. "The Microbiota and Health Promoting Characteristics of the Fermented Beverage Kefir." *Front Microbiol*, 2016 May.

Lamb, Jonathan. *The Rime of the Ancient Mariner, a Ballad of the Scurvy.* Clio Med. 2000 Princeton University Press, 2016.

Gates, Donna. *The Body Ecology Diet.* Atlanta: B.E.D. Publications, 1998.

Smith, Jeffrey. *Seeds of Deception.* Fairfield: Yes! Books, 2003.

Westgate, Megan. http://www.nongmoproject.org/learn-more/.

Delano, Maggie. http://web.mit.edu/demoscience/Monsanto/about.html. Spring 2009.

Paul, B., et al. "Influences of diet and the gut microbiome on epigenetic modulation in cancer and other diseases." *Clin Epigenetics*, 2015 Oct.

Lionetti, E., et al. "Gluten Psychosis: Confirmation of a New Clinical Entity." *Nutrients*, 2015 Jul.

Genuis, S., Lobo, R., et al. "Gluten Sensitivity Presenting as a Neuropsychiatric Disorder." *Gastroenterology Research and Practice*, Volume 2014, Article ID 293206.

Frankenfeld, C. "High-intensity sweetener consumption and gut microbiome content and predicted gene function in a cross-sectional study of adults in the United States." *Ann Epidemiol*, 2015 Oct.

Stoddard, Mary Nash. *The Deadly Deception*. Dallas: Compiled by the Aspartame Consumer Safety Network, 1996.

Vitetta, L., et al. "The gastrointestinal tract microbiome, probiotics, and mood." *Inflammopharmacology*, 2014 Dec.

Maes, M., Leunis, J. "Normalization of leaky gut in chronic fatigue syndrome (CFS) is accompanied by a clinical improvement: effects of age, duration of illness and the translocation of LPS from gram-negative bacteria." *Neuro Endocrinol Lett.* 2008 Dec.

Carradori, S., et al. "Antimicrobial activity, synergism and inhibition of germ tube formation by Crocus sativus-derived compounds against Candida spp." *J Enzyme Inhib Med Chem*, 2016 May.

Mazidi, M., et al. "A double-blind, randomized and placebo-controlled trial of Saffron (Crocus sativus L.) in the treatment of anxiety and depression." *J Complement Integr Med*, 2016 Jun.

Höfling, J., et al. "Antimicrobial potential of some plant extracts against Candida species." *Braz J Biol*, 2010 Nov.

Shen, J., et al. "Berberine up-regulates the BDNF expression in hippocampus and attenuates corticosterone-induced depressive-like behavior in mice." *Neurosci Lett*, 2016 Feb.

De Paula, L., et al. "Uncaria tomentosa (cat's claw) improves quality of life in patients with advanced solid tumors." *J Altern Complement Med*, 2015 Jan.

Qaseem, A., et al. "Nonpharmacologic Versus Pharmacologic Treatment of Adult Patients With Major Depressive Disorder: A Clinical Practice Guideline From the American College of Physicians." *Ann Intern Med*, 2016 Mar.

Süntar, I., et al. "Antimicrobial effect of the extracts from Hypericum perforatum against oral bacteria and biofilm formation." *Pharm Biol*, 2016 Jun.

Eck, Paul. *The Eck Institute of Applied Nutrition & Bioenergetics*, Ltd., Phoenix, AZ.

Donadio, G. "Organic vs. Non-Organically Grown Produce." *Rutgers University Study Posted in Nutrition*, 2012 Aug.

Bravoa, J. *Ingestion of Lactobacillus strain regulates emotional behavior and central GABA receptor expression in a mouse via the vagus nerve.* Edited by Todd R. Klaenhammer, North Carolina State University. Raleigh, NC. 2011 July.

Erasmus, Udo. *Fats that Heal, Fats that Kill.* Burnaby BC: Alive Books, 1986.

Chang, C., et al. "Essential fatty acids and human brain." *Acta Neurol Taiwan*, 2009 Dec.

Amminger, G., et al. "Longer-term outcome in the prevention of psychotic disorders by the Vienna omega-3 study." *Nat Commun*, 2015 Aug.

Hibbein, J., et al. "The potential for military diets to reduce depression, suicide, and impulsive aggression: a review of current evidence for omega-3 and omega-6 fatty acids." *Mil Med*, 2014 Nov.

Liu, J. et al. "Pathways of polyunsaturated fatty acid utilization: implications for brain function in neuropsychiatric health and disease." *Brain Res*, 2015 Feb.

Wu, A., et al. "Curcumin boosts DHA in the brain: Implications for the prevention of anxiety disorders." *Biochim Biophys Acta*, 2015 May.

Markhus, M. et al. "Docosahexaenoic Acid Status in Pregnancy Determines the Maternal Docosahexaenoic Acid Status 3-, 6- and 12 Months Postpartum. Results from a Longitudinal Observational Study." *PLoS One*, 2015 Sep.

Varteresian, T., et al. "Natural products and supplements for geriatric depression and cognitive disorders: an evaluation of the research." *Curr Psychiatry Rep*, 2014 Aug.

Yeap, S., et al. "Antistress and antioxidant effects of virgin coconut oil in vivo." *Exp Ther Med*, 2015 Jan.

Fernando, W., et al. "The role of dietary coconut for the prevention and treatment of Alzheimer's disease: potential mechanisms of action." *Br J Nutr*, 2015 Jul.

Hu Yang, I., et al. "Coconut Oil: Non-Alternative drug treatment against Alzheimer's disease." *Nutr Hosp*, 2015 Dec.

Shatzman, A., et al. "Gustin concentration changes relative to salivary zinc and taste in humans." *Proc Natl Acad Sci U S A.*, 1981 June.

Four-Week Personal Application Workbook

Gut Feelings

Unlocking Spiritual, Nutritional, and Intestinal Links to Anxiety, Depression & Fatigue

Introduction

It is impossible to write a book addressing the intricacies of health restoration which can then be applied to the unique facets of every single person. The cookie-cutter approach is not effective if your desire is to identify and rectify root cause issues for illness and disease. It is my hope that this Personal Application Workbook will personalize the various phases of this book to help you on your road to recovery. It is broken down into a weekly format—some weeks may require more time and commitment than others. Proceed at a pace that works for you.

Week One

Hope for Healing

Since the assumption is that you have read this book, it seems appropriate to begin the workbook at the end chapter which asks the question:

"Do you believe that God can heal you physically and emotionally?"

______Yes ______No

Hope is available to you, no matter what your current state of health.

Victimhood disempowers a person—this is what I call wilderness thinking. The Israelites turned what should have been an eleven day journey into forty years wandering around in the wilderness. The thought process of fear, rejection, shame and guilt becomes a vicious cycle if you stay steeped in victimhood, which is exactly what the enemy of your soul wants.

> *I have been crucified with Christ; and it is no longer I who live, but Christ lives in me, and the life which I now live in the flesh I live by faith in the Son of God, who loved me and gave Himself up for me.*
>
> Galatians 2:20

Wise choices are the fruit of knowledge. Hosea 4:6 says, "My people are destroyed for lack of knowledge." Your body can reverse the course of long-term illness and disease. Now the decision to seek optimal health, regardless of your diagnosis, rests with you.

Without faith, there is no hope. Not faith in a health care practitioner or a physician, or a drug or a supplement, but faith in the One God who created your entire being, your chemistry lab. No one knows your body better than you do, except Him. You can make the choice to take responsibility for the health of your beautiful body and mind. Then, and only then, will you be motivated, creating hope through God-appointed self-healing.

Prepare ahead of time. First Peter 1:13 instructs:

> *Therefore, prepare your minds for action, keep sober in spirit, fix your hope completely on the grace to be brought to you at the revelation of Jesus Christ.*

He peels, reveals and heals if you will allow Him! Let's move forward and see how!

Health the Way God Intended

Man & Machine

Unlike a hydraulic machine, God created your body in many miraculous ways, one of the most miraculous is to naturally seek healing. Pain is also given by God as a great motivator that the body uses to seek comfort or healing. For instance, a simple repositioning of your body after you have sat on your legs for too long a period of time. Or it can be applied to a frightening diagnosis of cancer after a routine colonoscopy. You either do something about it, or you ignore it.

Genesis, chapter 1, verse 27 states that, "God created man in His own image, in the image of God He created him; male and female He created them." He is pure and perfect, and He created us in His image to be pure and perfect. However, as the first of God's human creation, Adam's sin of disobedience in the garden caused an imperfect nature in each one of us. But, because of His incomparable grace and mercy we have the opportunity to once again conform to His image through His Son's shed blood on the cross. That is why Jesus came to earth.

Those who believe the following words spoken by Jesus in John 3:16 will have an eternally pure and perfect body.

> *For God so loved the world that He gave His only begotten Son, that whoever believes in Him shall not perish, but have eternal life.*

Your body must deal with variables on a constant basis in order to maintain homeostasis, or balance. List some of the variables your own body must deal with to try to maintain balance:

1. ______________________________
2. ______________________________
3. ______________________________
4. ______________________________
5. ______________________________
6. ______________________________

Oswald Chambers, says in his time-honored devotional, My Utmost for His Highest:

> "It is a fact that there is a continuing struggle in the physical, mental, moral, and spiritual areas of life. Health is the balance between the physical parts of my body and all the things and forces surrounding me. To maintain good health I must have sufficient internal strength to fight off the things that are external."

Signals & Alarms

First Peter 5:8 says, "Your adversary the devil prowls around like a roaring lion seeking someone to devour." Considering your state of health today, are you able to hear the enemy knocking on your door through your body's many whispers or cries for help? Beside each of the following signals and alarms, insert a "W" for a whisper (signal) for help or a "C" for a cry (alarm) for help:

______ Burping
______ Panic attacks
______ Painful and swollen joints
______ Abdominal cramping
______ Anxiousness
______ Fatigue
______ Exhaustion
______ Diarrhea
______ Constipation
______ Gas or bloating
______ Headaches
______ Reflux
______ Debilitating depression

Satan and his cohorts don't always knock. They barge in uninvited, or we invite them in through open doors of unhealthy lifestyle choices, whether those choices are fast food, lack of exercise, addictions to alcohol, sugar, drugs (including prescription drug abuse), smoking, spiritual bondages, or an otherwise unbalanced life. And that is right where the enemy wants you! It is so important to become familiar with your body. It is not necessary to become an expert in anatomy or physiology in order to recognize the signals and alarms (symptoms) that are your body's way of saying that all is not right. Every symptom is a God-given opportunity to find and fix what's wrong otherwise they become strongholds of the enemy.

Spiritual Strongholds

Spiritual bondages or strongholds are lies from the enemy which we have chosen to believe as truth either consciously or subconsciously. They create a wall or a barrier preventing you from becoming all that God has created you to be. Such a stronghold might be shame and guilt heaped on by the enemy over the years. Other bondages might be unforgiveness, anger and rejection—or lies that you're too fat, too skinny, too sick, not good enough, etc. The light of truth in the standard of God's word (the Bible) shines a light on these strongholds and identifies them for what they are—lies from the pit of hell, the home of the enemy of your soul.

Place a check mark beside any strongholds you may have already identified in your life preventing you from becoming all that God designed you to be:

______ Shame
______ Guilt
______ Anger
______ Fear
______ Unforgiveness
______ Bitterness
______ Rejection
______ Pride
______ ____________________

Bondages of all kinds were initiated in the Garden of Eden when Adam and Eve were disobedient to God's command to not eat from the tree of the knowledge of good and evil. Disobedience is what enslaves; obedience is what provides freedom. As the physical body heals, it remains critical that you remember the spiritual implications of ill health, which will be discussed further in Week Three.

Reversing Illness

Given the proper support, God created your body to heal itself. Your body strives for homeostasis, which is the state of all systems working properly. The sum total of a synergistically functioning body is more effective than each system working independently. However, your body systems do not work independently. Each requires input and feedback from the others, and no one body system is more important than another. Body systems and organs which become congested and toxic put stress and strain on other organs.

Insert a check beside each issue or body burden you may be dealing with and/or might be taking a pharmaceutical drug for:

______ Chronic respiratory issues
______ Chronic yeast infections
______ High blood pressure
______ Cravings
______ Lack of focus and concentration
______ Headaches/Migraines
______ Bladder/Kidney infections
______ Mood swings
______ High cholesterol or triglycerides
______ Unstable blood sugar/diabetes
______ Asthma or allergies
______ Indigestion
______ Depression
______ Anxiety
______ Joint/Muscle Pain
______ Premenstrual Symptoms
______ Fatigue

Treating symptoms with drugs can suppress the body's natural response, inhibit healing, and drive the disease or illness deeper into the cellular structure of the body. There is an alternative for almost every prescription drug available. In very few cases, the pharmaceutical approach may be the best temporary solution, but in others, you may be unnecessarily depositing toxins or interfering with the body's natural processes in order to treat symptoms that are easily alleviated with nutritional therapies. It is important to get to the root cause, which in most cases is directly related to the health of the gastrointestinal tract.

Your Divine Chemistry Lab

Think of your body as a chemistry lab designed and created by a Divine God. Every single thing you put into your body has a chemical effect whether you eat it, inhale it, think about it, or take it in through the skin. Every one of your other senses—sight, hearing, and touch, have an effect on your biochemistry, too. These biochemical reactions affect the body physically, emotionally and mentally potentially causing annoying symptoms such as those you checked earlier.

When you feed your body, you are either building health or promoting disease. Prolonged poor eating habits are capable of permanently altering your DNA. It would make sense, then, that each generation could become sicker and sicker. In other words, children are born with an already high body burden of toxins.

Long term poor food choices usher in more serious symptoms such as panic attacks, suicidal thoughts, obsessive-compulsive behavior, social phobias, mental confusion, violence, and aggressiveness. The prevalence of many types of so-called degenerative mental or emotional diseases including Alzheimer's and Parkinson's is an expression of the cellular hunger present in various states of malnutrition and toxicity.

Place a check mark beside any of the following which contributes to DNA gene alteration:

______ Environmental pollutants
______ Vaccinations
______ Additives, preservatives, colorings
______ Chemical sweeteners
______ Pesticides
______ Mineral oil
______ Plastics

______ Pharmaceutical and OTC drugs
______ Creams and lotions
______ "Beauty" injections
______ Negative thoughts and emotions

Gut

Scientifically speaking, the gut is the term for the alimentary canal (gastrointestinal tract) from the pyloric opening between the stomach and duodenum and the anus. The GI tract provides a barrier between itself and the internal environment of the rest of the body. It also provides surveillance by immune system tracking which determines the tolerance of all intestinal contents. As soon as it detects a substance as a foreign invader, the immune system (as an integral part of the gut) produces antibodies which grab onto the invaders in an attempt to make them less harmful.

The gastrointestinal tract, then, includes the stomach, small intestine, and large intestine. However, digestion and absorption accomplished through the GI could not be complete without the help of the brain, liver, gallbladder, pancreas, spinal column, central nervous system, immune system, lymphatic system and cardiovascular system. It is far more accurate to say that the entire body plays a part in digestion, absorption, and elimination.

Mouth & Digestion

Most of us have heard the phrase, "you are what you eat." The more physiologically accurate phrase is, "you are what you ______ ________, ___________, ___________ and _________________." Digestion begins in the __________________.

Stomach

Food travels from the mouth through the esophagus to the stomach. The pH of the stomach should be approximately "1" on the pH scale, which is very acidic. A drop of stomach acid (hydrochloric acid or Hcl) can eat through the paint on your car.

Acid in the stomach is necessary (answer true or false):

______ To kill bacteria and other pathogens
______ To breakdown food entering from the esophagus
______ It is not necessary—that is why acid-blockers were discovered

If the stomach produces insufficient hydrochloric acid and does not have the enzyme and bile support of the liver, gallbladder, and pancreas to break down protein, carbohydrates and fat, the food contents will sit in the stomach longer than necessary and putrefy and ferment. This gaseous production will cause the valve from the stomach to the esophagus to open moving bile acids into the esophagus.

Proton pump inhibitors (PPI) and H2 blockers prescribed for heartburn and GERD inhibit the absorption of Vitamin B12 which can cause pernicious anemia, dementia, and will also interfere with liver methylation.

Methylation

Methylation is one of the many pathways in the liver that helps to detoxify, convert and contribute to a wide range of critical body functions. Methylation is considered among scientists as a critical epigenetic process, having serious health implications, which include mental and emotional dysfunction. At the same time, improvements in the function of this pathway can show substantial improvement in overall health. Symptoms that this pathway may not be working might be irritability, mood swings, anxiety, fatigue, estrogen excess, or gallbladder issues.

Methylation defects may contribute to major chronic conditions. Place a check mark next to any of the following that you may be dealing with:

______ Mood and psychiatric disorders such as anxiety, depression, bi-polar disorder, schizophrenia
______ Fatigue
______ Addictive behaviors

______ Cardiovascular disease
______ Cancer
______ Diabetes
______ Alzheimer's disease
______ Seizures
______ Autoimmune disorders
______ Premature aging
______ Infertility, miscarriage and pregnancy issues
______ Autism and other neurospectrum disorders
______ Lyme disease

Most all of us think of complications within the brain when considering Alzheimer's disease. While that is true, consider also that depleted vitamin B12 prevents proper methylation in the liver pathway, and it will indirectly affect the brain with the potential for depression, fatigue, and anxiety, as well. A by-product of the methylation cycle in the liver is an amino acid called homocysteine. If this chemical becomes too high (easily measured in blood), it will affect long-term cognitive function.

You should know your levels of at least the following tests in order to know how well your liver methylation pathway is working:

Homocysteine, serum – level should be 4.5 – 8.0. Your level is: ____________________

Vitamin B12, serum – level should be 750 – 1200. Your level is: ________________________

MTHFR (methyltetrahydrofolate-reductase), cheek swab to check for genetic defect. Your level is: _____________

Small and Large Intestine

The small and large intestine make up the largest terrain of the immune system. They are home to almost four pounds, or about one-hundred trillion and four-hundred different species of good and bad bacteria. These bacteria must be balanced, are critical to the health of the gastrointestinal tract, and necessary as a preventive model for almost every disease process.

Place a check mark next to some responsibilities of bacteria in the gut:

______ Consume the waste from the foods you eat
______ Disable toxic materials
______ Make vitamins
______ Key helper for the immune system
______ Produce short chain fatty acids for gut protection
______ Provide for delivery of information to the brain
______ Get your slippers

True or False?

______ The small intestine is about five-feet in length and about one-inch in diameter.

______ The large intestine is about twenty-feet in length and about two and one-half inches in diameter.

It is important that the transit time, or the time it takes between eating a food and eliminating the waste products from that food, is between eighteen and twenty-six hours. Less than twelve hours is too fast and not a long enough time period for proper absorption. More than twenty-six hours the waste begins to putrefy, ferment, and even cling to the intestinal wall.

Track your own transit time. At any time, swallow the contents of one tablespoon sesame seeds, which can be mixed with food or drink. Mark the day and time, then note the day and time that you first notice sesame seeds in the stool. Your transit time is ____ ______________ hours.

It is throughout this entire length of the gastrointestinal tract that damage and inflammation can occur, including destroying mucus where mucus should be or creating mucus where mucus should not be. Accumulated toxic waste as well as bacteria, fungus, virus, and other pathogens, begin the pattern of functional disease causing signals or whispers for help such as constipation, diarrhea, gas, bloating, heartburn, GERD, and belching. If this path is allowed to continue, declining physical health is inevitable including the soul sicknesses of anxiety, depression, and fatigue.

Acute or chronic symptoms that you experience now or have in the past which you think might be related to your gut health:

1. ______________________________
2. ______________________________
3. ______________________________
4. ______________________________
5. ______________________________
6. ______________________________
7. ______________________________
8. ______________________________
9. ______________________________
10. ______________________________

Week Two

What Causes a Toxic Body?

Harmful metabolites that cannot be converted or moved out of the body get stored in tissue structures of the body like joints, muscles, nerves, bones, etc. A toxic gastrointestinal tract is a favorable environment for parasites, fungus, yeast, bad bacteria, virus and other organisms to build and prosper. As these organisms feast on the fermented and putrefied food, end-products in the intestinal terrain, they create their own metabolic waste, which further burdens the body's detoxification processes.

Liver & Gall-Bladder Inefficiencies

A healthy functioning liver and gallbladder are challenged by pregnancy, gallstones, alcohol abuse, anabolic steroids, and various chemicals or drugs, including birth control pills. One of the liver's key jobs, through its methylation pathway, is to covert and properly dismantle estrogen, otherwise excess estrogen can also cause thickness of the bile leading to gallstones. Not just the hormone estrogen, but estrogen mimics, also called xenoestrogens, can be found in meats, dairy products, plastics, pollutants, pesticides and body lotions and creams. These substances look like estrogen to the body and the liver tries to process them as such, further burdening the process of detoxification and creating hormone imbalance.

Even if you ingest a good diet, you may still have more toxins than the body's systems can handle. We are exposed to many body burdens on an on-going basis. Insert a check beside each one that is a part of your dietary intake or lifestyle:

______ Pesticides or herbicides
______ Antibiotics
______ Food additives, preservatives, and colorings
______ Birth control pills or steroids
______ Chemical sweeteners
______ Hormones
______ Nicotine
______ Excessive caffeine

______ Drugs
______ Vaccinations
______ Prescription and over-the-counter drugs
______ Body lotions, shampoos, cream and potions

Bowel Elimination

The sluggish colon has an enormous capacity to collect waste. The collected waste, over time, becomes rigidly attached to the wall of the colon just like pappier-mache hardens, where it releases additional toxins into the body and prevents proper absorption of nutrients. How many bowel movements do you have daily on a consistent basis?

__________ times daily or weekly

The solution to pollution is dilution. Water is absolutely essential to all body functions. How many ounces of purified water do you drink daily on a consistent basis?

__________ ounces

Leaky-Gut Syndrome

This particular aspect of gastrointestinal links to recovery from anxiety, depression and fatigue is a term which refers to small and large intestine permeability or, more accurately, hyper-permeability. Complex protein structures called "tight junctions" are responsible for maintaining the seal of the entire intestinal tract.

When these intestinal barriers become compromised, toxins as well as other substances like partially digested food particles can penetrate the intestinal wall and leak into the bloodstream. These microscopic particles then circulate through the body and cause a number of symptoms, most notably food allergies and asthma. However, this gut hyper-permeability can cause the immune system itself to be confused and destroy the body's own cells, manifesting in any number of autoimmune diseases.

The easiest way to know if you have "leaky-gut" is simply based on your symptoms. Place a check mark beside any of these symptoms which apply to you. The number you check gives you a clue as to the degree of permeability:

______ Fatigue or exhaustion
______ Depression
______ Anxiety or panic attacks
______ Chronic use of medications, aspirin, acetaminophen, NSAIDS, corticosteroids, antibiotics
______ Poor diet, including alcohol excess
______ Infections from parasites, virus, bacteria, or fungus
______ Gut problems like GERD, IBS, IBD, gas, bloating, constipation, or diarrhea
______ Food sensitivities, allergies, or asthma
______ Chronic insomnia or sleeplessness
______ Autoimmune diseases such as eczema, psoriasis, Lupus, Hashimoto's thyroiditis, arthritis, etc.

This list hardly excludes anyone, right? This gut permeation can be healed, but it takes time, the right dietary intake, and the right cleansing and re-building programs.

Sources of Toxic Burden

Generally and simplistically speaking there are three basic reasons for a toxic body: burden from foreign pathogens, an unprotected body, and an inefficient detoxification system.

1. Antibiotics

Antibiotics kill not only the bad bacteria, but the good as well, altering the balance of protective gut flora and immunity defense. The immune system in the gut has been left unprotected, compromised and incapable of defending the body against invasion.

2. Fungal Overgrowth

Place a check mark beside any of the following fungus-related symptoms which you may experience:

______ Brain fog/Poor Memory
______ Sugar and carbohydrate cravings
______ Fatigue, anxiety, depression
______ Vaginal yeast infection/jock itch
______ Fingernail or toenail fungus
______ Rashes, eczema, other skin problems
______ Premenstrual tension
______ Tinnitus
______ Bloating, belching, intestinal gas
______ Mucous in the stool
______ Chronic respiratory issues
______ Easy bruising

3. Parasites

Parasites and fungus usually populate together and typically reside in the GI tract. Yet, as with fungus, parasites can build a nest anywhere in the body. Check any of the following signs and symptoms of a parasitic infection which may apply to you:

______ Rectal itching and/or pressure
______ Diarrhea
______ Mucous in stools and poorly formed stools
______ Muscular wasting and/or weakness
______ Chronic vague abdominal pain with constant belching
______ Ravenous appetite
______ Constant or frequent heartburn after eating
______ Bloating after eating, especially digestive distress after eating fatty foods
______ Unexplained weight loss or inability to gain weight
______ Night sweats and insomnia
______ Itchy skin, worse at night
______ Chronic dark circles under the eyes

4. Virus & Bacteria

Virus and bacteria are other foreign invaders which will compromise the terrain of the gut and the entire body. Most notably are helicobacter pylori, E.coli, salmonella, campylobacter, listeria, clostridium, and streptococcus. Virus and bacteria not only cause damage physically, but mentally as well.

5. Heavy Metals & Other Destructive Chemicals

Our world today is bombarded with old and newly created harmful chemicals which surround us even from the moment of conception. They're in our face cleansers, toothpaste, shower soap, shampoo, make-up, body lotions and potions, plastics, clothing, car materials, furniture, not to mention the food we eat and the air we breathe. They obstruct the body's Divinely-orchestrated dance of hormones within the brain, the organs and glands, and the central nervous system.

6. Stressors

Yes, stressors are sources of toxins. It's not the stressor itself, but the thoughts we think about these stressors. The thoughts, whether negative or positive about finances, jobs, time management, family or marriage, and social values all produce biochemical reactions that affect our health. Stressors are energy wasters and, as such, upset biochemical balance. Negative emotions relating to these stressors become part of the biochemical make-up of organs and systems.

Of the above (or other) stressors, choose the one that causes you the most stress. Now, write down all your thoughts about it. Underline the positive ones and circle the negative ones.

Biggest Stressor: ______________________________

My thoughts about it: ______________________________

____

____

____

____

____

____

____

____

7. Poor Dietary Intake

Refer to pages 119 and 120 and list below any Bad-Mood Foods that you regularly consume:

1. ______________________________
2. ______________________________
3. ______________________________
4. ______________________________
5. ______________________________
6. ______________________________
7. ______________________________
8. ______________________________

Anxiety & Depression are Not All in Your Head

The Effect of Food on Mood

An entire cascade of biochemical reactions occurs when food is ingested. Your entire body and psychoemotional system become involved.

Which of the following emotions have you experienced in relation to lack of food?

______ Anxiety or panic
______ Fatigue, sleepiness or lethargy
______ Jitteriness (external or internal)
______ Anger or irritability
______ Aggressiveness
______ Rage

Neurotransmitters Role in Food & Mood

Neurotransmitters are chemicals which participate in the communication when food is digested and absorbed. Serotonin, dopamine, GABA, epinephrine, norepinephrine are the primary neurotransmitters involved—they are tied to emotional reactions, as well.

Any of the following issues can relate to neurotransmitter imbalances caused by disturbances in the gut. Place "A" (acute), or "C" (chronic) beside any of the following issues which you experience:

______ Anxiety or panic attacks
______ Depression/Bipolar disorder
______ Poor digestion, including gas and bloating
______ Carbohydrate and sugar cravings
______ Headaches
______ Insomnia
______ Hot flashes
______ Addictions and cravings
______ Lethargy or fatigue
______ Sleeping too much
______ Feelings of immobility
______ Lack of motivation
______ Procrastination

The Role of Adrenal Fatigue in Anxiety & Depression

In recent years cortisol, which is a primary hormone produced by the adrenals, has been continually disparaged as a "bad" hormone. Nothing could be farther from the truth. Cortisol is critical to life playing the starring role in the body's stress response. Cortisol does become an issue, however, when it is forced to work overtime and results in imbalanced health.

The following are potential sources of stress which increase the demand for cortisol.

Place a check mark next to any that you experience now or have in the past:

______ Feelings of inadequate digestion
______ Whiplash and other head trauma
______ Inflammation and pain
______ Prolonged temperature extremes
______ Toxic exposures to chemicals, and radiation
______ Infections
______ Negative emotions like anger, guilt, shame, worry, or fear

______ Anxiety and depression
______ Workaholism
______ Sleep deprivation

Over time, chronically elevated cortisol will manifest symptoms such as anxiety, panic attacks, fatigue, and depression, especially in the presence of digestive issues and neurotransmitter imbalance. Chronically high cortisol output by the adrenals will eventually result in adrenal burnout with symptoms including exhaustion, cognitive dysfunction, anxiety, and depression.

Do you have Adrenal Burn-out?

The principal physical symptom that initially identifies burnout is overwhelming fatigue upon awakening in the morning or after a brief nap. In short, the individual feels exhausted. Place a check mark beside any of the following symptoms of adrenal burn out which you may experience:

______ Depletion of progesterone, testosterone, and other hormones
______ Protein and fat malabsorption
______ Decrease in lean muscle mass
______ Sick more than one time per year
______ Low or high blood sugar
______ Chronic inflammation or pain
______ Poor memory or concentration
______ Foggy thoughts
______ Depression
______ Anxiety and worry
______ Feelings of guilt or shame
______ Exhaustion
______ Sense of being overwhelmed
______ Insomnia or poor sleep
______ Headaches
______ Heart palpitations
______ Low libido
______ Cold hands and feet

______ Inability to lose weight
______ Chronic low blood pressure
______ Back pain or tight neck and shoulders
______ Muscle twitching
______ Digestive/bowel issues
______ Chronic infections, including skin rashes

If you placed a check mark beside eight or more symptoms, you are likely experiencing adrenal burnout.

Physical, Spiritual & Emotional Recovery from Burnout

Your physical, emotional, and spiritual health are intertwined and function without separation throughout the framework of your body, soul and spirit.

It is critical to reduce known stressors where you can and to recreate your attitude toward those that are not in your control. Stressors can relate to fear of failure, fear of not having enough, fear of sickness and pain, fear of rejection or abandonment, or fear of not being protected. Many of these can relate to spiritual bondages from as far back as when you were in the womb.

Stress almost always involves fear and the antidote to fear is always faith. Not faith itself, but in whom the faith is placed. In order to have faith, you have to believe and trust in what or whom your faith is placed. That Person is the one, true God. Faith in Him to do what He says He will do. Know Him by reading His revealed truth in the Bible. If you ask Him and trust Him, He will wipe away all your fears. Your life may not be perfect, but He has a plan for your perfection.

List those things which you feel are stressors in your life:

1. ______
2. ______
3. ______
4. ______
5. ______
6. ______

Circle those stressors that don't line up with who God created you to be and your goal of recovery. Of those that remain, reduce or delegate the least important ones.

Make another list, writing down what is most important to you:

1. ____
2. ____
3. ____
4. ____
5. ____
6. ____

Eliminate those things or relationships with people in your life which don't line up with your purpose in life. Recreate your attitude by acknowledging that you are not responsible for the operation of the world. The world is God's responsibility and He is in control. Your responsibility is to listen, obey, and be still and know that He is God (Psalm 46:10). Allow God to change and restore you through His great mercy and grace.

Week Three

The Inflammatory Role in Depression and Anxiety

Psychological stress impairs the body's ability to regulate inflammation and can promote the development and progression of disease. The immune system is compromised during times of stress causing minor "routine" illnesses, which then lay a tragic foundation for more debilitating diseases like lupus, CFIDS (chronic fatigue immune dysfunction syndrome), fibromyalgia, rheumatoid arthritis, and others.

Insert a check mark beside any of the following so-called routine illnesses (underlying root causes), and debilitating diseases which you have had or are currently experiencing:

______ Chronic respiratory infections
______ Asthma/allergies
______ Arthritis
______ Poor diet
______ Intestinal bowel diseases
______ Headaches
______ Plantar fasciitis
______ Skin rashes
______ Constipation
______ Diarrhea
______ Kidney or Gall Stones
______ Depression
______ Anxiety
______ Colon cancer
______ Hormone-related cancers (breast, prostate, ovarian, uterine, etc.)

The vagus nerve provides two-way communication from the brain to the gut and back. For every one nerve fiber sending messages from the brain to the gut, there are nine which return messages and information from the gut to the brain.

The gut-brain axis does provide a breakthrough for hope through the recognition that you were created by God and you work as a whole being: spirit, soul, and body. Not one system or part of your being can operate exclusively, but they synergistically support one another physically, emotionally, and spiritually in the body's on-going attempt to maintain health or perpetuate healing.

This model of disease process for anxiety, depression, and fatigue also gives hope to the individual suffering. Being guided by the whole being and root cause model also persuades against applying a bandage antidepressant or anti-anxiety prescription without uncovering the real cause of these psychological symptoms.

List any antidepressant, anti-anxiety, or other medication you were prescribed where the physician did not discuss dietary intake or any other potential root causes.

1. ______________________________
2. ______________________________
3. ______________________________
4. ______________________________

Thyroid Inflammation

Dysregulation of either the thyroid or adrenal glands can certainly lead to mental or emotional symptoms, as well as many other concerns. As with the adrenal glands, the thyroid gland is also controlled by the hypothalamus and the pituitary glands in the cranial cavity, so it is referred to as the HPT axis.

Do you suffer from any of these common symptoms of low thyroid, even though your physician told you your thyroid is "normal?" Insert a check mark beside each one that applies:

______ Cold hands and feet
______ Constipation
______ Fatigue
______ Infertility
______ Weight gain
______ Joint & muscle aches and pains
______ Lethargy
______ Lack of focus or concentration/memory

______ Depression
______ Dry skin
______ Hair loss
______ Sleeping too much
______ Insomnia

Restoring Mental and Emotional Health through the Gut Highway

Detoxification to Prevent Foundational Stages of Disease

Cleansing & Detoxification

Fill in the blanks:

____________________ refers to a flushing out of loose waste material and is most often related to the large bowel (colon). This can be accomplished in a couple of days. ________________, however, is a complete supplemental nutritional protocol which lasts anywhere from ten to thirty days (longer for those with more serious chronic issues).

Detoxification and cleansing are generally accomplished at the same time during this time-frame. The goal is to upregulate or optimize those systems of the body which are involved in this natural day-to-day process.

The following is an abbreviated list of symptoms that indicate the body is burdened with toxic material and that cleansing or detoxification would be beneficial. Place a check mark beside any that you experience:

______ Digestive complaints of any kind
______ Depression
______ Anxiety and panic attacks
______ Fatigue, lethargy
______ Arthritis and other auto-immune illnesses

______ Body odor or bad breath
______ Insomnia
______ Headaches
______ Low back pain
______ Poor memory or concentration
______ Sciatica
______ Asthma and allergies
______ Chronic colds, flu, bronchitis
______ Any disease process

Based on your responses, on the following continuum, place an "X" where you believe your health falls:

Healthy	A few pesky signals	More than a few signals	Many chronic issues

The body heals in reverse chronological order, so it heals the cold you had last week before it heals the mononucleosis you had in college, and before it heals the pneumonia you had as a child. It also heals from the inside out, so it heals a leaky gut before the final healing stages of a skin disorder. The healing of the physical body will be accelerated through spiritual healing and recovery led by the Holy Spirit, who gives hope because of our faith in Him as the Healer.

> *For he will be like a tree planted by the water that extends its roots by a stream, and* ***will not fear*** *when the heat comes; but its leaves will be green, and it* ***will not be anxious*** *in a year of drought nor cease to yield fruit (emphasis mine).*
>
> Jeremiah 17:8

Periodic detoxification is important for an optimally functioning body and one of the best proactive steps you can take to expedite balanced physical and mental health. Trees are no better than their root system, and so it is with your body—you are no healthier than your root system, the 'terrain' of your gut.

Exit Pathway Clearance

It is important to follow cellular detoxification in a step process to prevent becoming even sicker than you might have been when you started. Even if you feel healthy, toxins deposited at the cellular level may not yet have created initial symptoms, and you might still become sick during the initial process. Put the following six-steps in order (you may refer back to pages 99-100):

______ Add support for liver and gallbladder detoxification
______ Support the immune system
______ Support to kill and rid the body of yeast and fungus, virus, bacteria, parasites, heavy metals, and chemicals
______ Be sure the lymph and colon are up-regulated to function properly
______ Change your dietary intake to remove harmful or interference foods.
______ Make sure other exit pathways such as the skin, the kidneys, and the respiratory system are open and clearing properly

Spiritual Roots that Impede Physical and Emotional Healing

Addressing spiritual strongholds always helps to expedite physical and emotional healing when carried out at the same time. Cleansing and detoxification is an amazing picture of how the Heavenly Father peels, reveals, and heals, not only from a physiological perspective, but also on a mental and emotional level.

Identifying and releasing spiritual bondages—a kind of nutrition for the soul—is the most important step in a complete health restoration process. You are a spiritual being in a physical body with a soul. The soul consists of mind, will, and emotions and, thereby, has thoughts, makes choices and has feelings.

The thoughts you think and the emotions you feel (especially negative) can overburden your system on a cellular level. Each thought and emotion, whether negative or positive, has a biochemical response which must be metabolized by the body's organs and systems of detoxification. Unresolved emotions wound deeply, forming harmful chemical byproducts which, if the body cannot get rid of, get stored in the cellular tissue creating what we might call soul sicknesses of anxiety and depression.

Byproducts of negative emotions increase acid in the body causing disease at the cellular level. Even cancer in the early stages is a silent inflammatory disease process that impedes cellular communication.

Place a check mark beside any of the following issues which you feel might be a stronghold of the enemy for you personally:

______	Anger	_________	Guilt
______	Fear	_________	Rejection
______	Bitterness	_________	Pride
______	Shame	_________	Unforgiveness

Consider by asking the Holy Spirit to reveal to you how these strongholds cause you to see yourself and how they are interfering with your health, your relationship with others, and your relationship with Jesus Christ. Write in the blank space below. Take your time and do not rush what the Holy Spirit wants to reveal. Use a journal or another sheet of paper, if necessary.

Emotions Get Stored

When natural detoxification processes are overburdened, the chemical byproducts of toxic thoughts and emotions get stored in various organs, glands and systems of the body. Left unchecked and allowed to fester, these become forms of spiritual bondage. Cleansing, detoxification, and spiritual healing programs clear up congestion in these pathways allowing electrical energy to once again flow unimpeded.

Fill in the blanks, choosing from: liver, gallbladder, kidneys, pancreas, small intestine, large intestine, stomach, respiratory system, lungs, skin, and heart (you may refer back to pages 105-106):

Bitterness is stored in the ______________________.

Anger, frustration, jealously, and envy are stored in the _____ ______________________ and ______________________.

Grief, hate, and impatience are stored in the ______________ and small ______________________.

Fear is stored in the ______________________ system and ______________________________.

Worry, anxiety, and mistrust are stored in the ____________ and ________________.

Guilt, shame, and depression are stored in ______________, ________________ and large ________________.

Anger is almost always a secondary emotion. The primary emotion might be fear, and the spiritual root of fear might be abandonment. The antidote to fear of any kind is always faith... not in faith itself, but the object of that faith—the only One in whom you can ultimately place your trust—Jesus Christ. A Christian counselor can help identify the deeper spiritual root which will expedite the body to respond to healing protocols. Additionally, time spent through journaling and interaction with the Holy Spirit of Jesus Christ who is the greatest Counselor and Healer will help you recreate your road to personal health.

He longs to show you all things. Trust Him to peel back the layers for you physically and emotionally, to reveal what He wants you to know, and to be healed according to His perfect timing. Addressing revolving negative thoughts and emotions will support a framework for making God-intended choices and allow you to hear His voice more clearly.

Second Corinthians 10:5 says to take every thought captive. Capture and trap those negative thoughts, wrap them in a garbage bag like the trash they are, and destroy them.

> *We are destroying speculations and every lofty thing raised up against the knowledge of God, and we are taking every thought captive to the obedience of Christ.*

If at any time, you feel overwhelmed physically or emotionally, stop the cleanse process, grab a journal and begin asking and recording what it is that God wants to reveal to you. As He peels, He reveals and heals. This is an excellent opportunity to spend time building your relationship with Christ.

Week Four

Restoring Digestive Function

With the exception of releasing spiritual bondages, restoring the gastrointestinal tract is perhaps the most critical step in any quest for health. Enzymes are required for clearing and rebuilding, as well as necessary for every single function in the body including digesting, absorbing, transporting, metabolizing, and eliminating the waste of foods from the diet.

Review the Chart of Enzyme Relationships on page 113-114 and check below those you feel relate to any health issues you may have:

______ Amylase
______ Lipase
______ Cellulose
______ Sucrose
______ Lactase
______ Maltase
______ Proteolytic enzymes
______ Hydrochloric acid (Hcl)

Dietary Changes for Recovery and Locked-In Healing

Dietary intake is extremely important to rebuilding gut health. Your body is a chemistry lab. The food you eat creates mixtures of chemical responses that affect our bodies in either healthful or harmful ways.

Food is, of course, a necessity—it's not only the fuel on which your body runs, it's also necessary to replenish, for recovery, and for restoration. Since your body requires an array of different vitamins, minerals, amino acids, fats, protein, carbohydrates and other nutrients, it needs a variety of different foods to meet those requirements. A monotonous diet doesn't meet these needs.

Think about your dietary intake on a regular basis. List four-six staple foods that you eat five-seven times per week (in other words, how monotonous is your diet?):

1. ______________________________
2. ______________________________
3. ______________________________
4. ______________________________
5. ______________________________
6. ______________________________

Food and Psychology

In our society today, food and drink have many uses. Insert a check mark beside any of the following reasons you might consume a particular food:

______ Numb painful memories
______ Anger
______ Fear
______ Depression
______ Rejection
______ Loneliness
______ Anxiousness
______ Fatigue

Now list three or four foods which you usually turn to or crave during those times:

1. ______________________________
2. ______________________________
3. ______________________________
4. ______________________________

Food addictions and abuses such as binge eating, anorexia, and bulimia very commonly have psychological as well as physiological and spiritual associations. Your thoughts and word choices about your behaviors also affect how your body responds. Constantly using negative words about self-behavior are not profitable for healing. What are some defeating thoughts and word choices the flesh, the enemy, or the world uses to mess with your mind:

1. ______________________________
2. ______________________________
3. ______________________________
4. ______________________________
5. ______________________________
6. ______________________________

List the proper response to these attacks: ________________
____

Regard your body as a temple where the Holy Spirit of God resides (1 Corinthians 3:16). Keep your temple clean and pure physically, mentally and spiritually.

It is important to realize emotional connections to eating, but to realize, also, that Satan and his demons want nothing more than to mess with your mind and to convince you that you will never be good enough, you will never overcome your addictions, or any number of other crushing and conquering words which continue to beat down. In order for the healing process to continue, you must realize that God is your victorious warrior, and that He has ultimate power.

Good-Mood and Bad-Mood Foods

For a minimum of six weeks eliminate the bad-mood foods listed on pages 119-120, and of the good-mood foods listed on pages 120-121 you may eat until content—but not full. On the following pages, keep a daily food diary, including any range of emotions felt each day. Be sure to have protein for breakfast, lunch, and dinner, and if you are experiencing symptoms of adrenal burnout follow the protocol under the section: *Dietary Changes—When Willpower Isn't Enough* on page 79. These food diary pages can be easily copied, or you may choose a separate journal. Use what works for you.

Food & Mood Diary

Date	Time	Food Eaten	Reason

Rebuilding with Micronutrient Supplementation

Supplements are just what the name implies—to supplement a dietary food intake with the necessary nutrition for the body to remain stable or increase in health. The reasons for nutrient deficiencies are many. Place a check mark beside any issues that may apply to you personally:

______ Stress
______ Antibiotic intake
______ Genetic defects
______ Poor diet
______ Good diet
______ Chemicals
______ Preservatives
______ Prescription and non-Rx drugs
______ Laxatives
______ Adrenal burnout
______ Low thyroid
______ Any diagnosed illness or disease
______ Other ______________________

Vitamins

Nutrients in the body are like dominoes standing on end in a neat little row several feet in length. Gently tapping the first one causes the entire row to cascade perfectly. Now remove one here and there. The "cascade" will never be accomplished properly because of the missing dominoes. So vitamins and minerals depend on one another to carry out the many cascades of metabolic and chemical activities that must occur in the body to provide optimal health.

Study the water-soluble and fat-soluble vitamin charts on pages 134-136. List the nutrients which you feel may be deficient in your own body:

1. ______________________________
2. ______________________________
3. ______________________________
4. ______________________________
5. ______________________________
6. ______________________________

Minerals

Vitamins cannot function without minerals, and mineral imbalances in the body are a key factor for a poor microbiome as well as energy depletion. Vitamins are like the gas in your car, and minerals are like the spark plugs which ignite the fuel. Minerals are uniquely involved in your body's ability to feel emotion. Every mineral has a reflective effect on mental and emotional health and, thereby, expressly linked to anxiety, depression and fatigue.

Study the mineral chart on pages 140-141. List below the minerals in which you feel you may be deficient:

1. ______________________________
2. ______________________________
3. ______________________________
4. ______________________________
5. ______________________________
6. ______________________________

Essential Amino Acids

Amino acids are critical for enzyme function, and enzymes, as we've already seen, are critical for every single activity in the human body. Nine of the twenty-one are essential, meaning the body cannot make them—we must get them from an outside source. Which of the following are the best sources of amino acids?

_____ Protein shakes
_____ Beef
_____ Fruits & veggies
_____ Granola bar
_____ Chicken
_____ Bagels
_____ Donuts
_____ Eggs

Because amino acids support the production of neurotransmitters, they should always be considered as part of a natural health program to relieve fatigue and reverse depression and anxiety. Study the amino acid chart on page 143. List below any in which you feel you may be deficient:

1. ______________________________
2. ______________________________
3. ______________________________

Essential Fatty Acids

Eating the right kinds of fats is not only part of a successful recovery package for depression, anxiety and fatigue, but is absolutely critical to life. A membrane composed of lipids (fats) surrounds every cell in the body. Essential fatty acids (EFAs) are a critical component of these membranes. Your body needs fatty acids to (check all that apply):

______ Digest
______ Dismantle and eliminate toxins
______ Generate energy
______ Support immune system
______ Support brain function
______ Alleviate pain and inflammation
______ Weight loss
______ Eliminate cravings

Place a check mark beside healthy dietary fats that should be included in your diet:

______ Avocados
______ Babe's fried chicken
______ Seeds & nuts
______ Coconut oil
______ Fish & their oils
______ Partially hydrogenated oils
______ Corn-fed beef
______ Olive oil
______ Organic butter
______ French fries
______ Margarine
______ Hydrogenated oils

General Recommendations for Bloodwork and other Testing Guidelines

General blood work at a local lab is a good start; however, it does not show a functional disease process—only a disease which has already manifested itself, or not. And, results from blood work can be quite misleading when it comes to nutritional status—even cancer patients have reported perfect blood work.

It is necessary to look at the function of the body from many different angles with an eye to root cause. An early warning report can be gathered from other nutritional screenings such as those listed on pages 147-151. Then, from the testing guidelines, choose those which you feel may be appropriate for you. Wisdom from God's Word in Jeremiah 31:21a instructs that we should:

> *"Set up for yourself road marks, place for yourself guideposts; direct your mind to the highway, the way by which you go."*

To determine which tests you may need, think about and answer the following:

- Family history
- Your previous history, including current diagnosis
- Genetic markers
- Functional disease processes based on signals and alarms which you have learned from this book
- Your personal history of dietary intake
- Any supplements you currently take
- Prescription and over-the-counter drugs you take or were recommended to take

Then, from the testing guidelines on pages 147-151, choose those which you feel may be appropriate for you.

About the Author

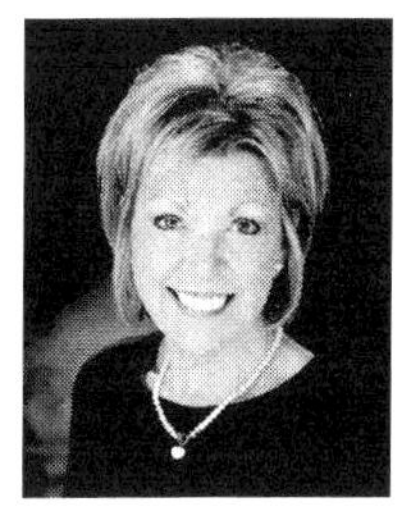

Dr. Sharon R. Price is a skilled clinician and a passionate research scientist. She founded Nutritional Direction in the Dallas/Ft. Worth area in January 1996, and has guided thousands of individuals on their health journey. As her first course of study, she received the Certified Nutritionist designation from American Health Science University. Sharon earned a Doctorate in Physiology in Natural Health Science, as well as her undergraduate Bachelor's and Master's in Nutrition from Clayton College of Natural Health. Dr. Price is also a Certified Bioenergetic Practitioner focusing on health as it relates to energy meridian pathways in the body.

In addition to keynote presentations, media appearances, and contributions to various natural health and community publications, Dr. Price has published two previous books, *Health & the Domino Effect* and *Culinary Creativity.*

She can be contacted at her direct email address:

drprice@nutritionaldirection.com.